Medical Emergencies
Diagnosis and Management

Medical Emergencies
Diagnosis and Management

FIFTH EDITION

RICHARD ROBINSON

FRCP
formerly Registrar to the Renal Unit, Guy's Hospital,
London

ROBIN STOTT

MA, FRCP
Consultant Physician, Lewisham Hospital, Lewisham

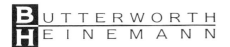

Butterworth-Heinemann Ltd
Linacre House, Jordan Hill, Oxford OX2 8DP

 PART OF REED INTERNATIONAL BOOKS

OXFORD   LONDON   BOSTON
MUNICH   NEW DELHI   SINGAPORE   SYDNEY
TOKYO   TORONTO   WELLINGTON

First published 1970
Second edition 1976
Reprinted with revisions 1977
Reprinted 1979
Third edition 1980
Reprinted 1981
Fourth edition 1983
Reprinted 1985, 1986
Fifth edition 1987
Reprinted 1989 (twice), 1991, 1992

British Library Cataloguing in Publication Data
Robinson, Richard
  Medical emergencies: diagnosis and
  management—5th ed.
  1. Emergency medicine
  I. Title   II. Stott, Robin
  616'.025   RC86.7

ISBN 0 7506 0274 0

Printed and bound in Great Britain by
Thomson Litho Ltd, East Kilbride, Scotland

Contents

Acknowledgements

Cardiovascular	Graham Jackson
Respiratory	John Rees and Carol Wengraf
Gastrointestinal	Gordon Sladen
Renal	Chisholm Ogg
Endocrine	Harry Keen
Neurology	Richard Hughes
The overdose	Tim Meredith
General	Gordon Jackson
Psychiatric and social problems	Derry McDiarmid
Closed head injury	Charles Polkey

Also the long suffering Mrs Sue Case and Mrs Marian Denney for
their secretarial help.

Foreword

Every well-educated, newly appointed, pre-registration house officer on the way to answer a call to deal with a medical emergency experiences the same anxieties about his ability to discharge his responsibilities when he gets there. One of my own strong memories is set in the casualty room at Johns Hopkins where I was acting as a locum intern: I recall a more senior colleague—long since an eminent professor of medicine—reaching up to take bottles of sterile glucose from the shelf as the comatose (hypoglycaemic) patient was wheeled in on the ambulance trolley. How could one, I wondered, ever match this speedy diagnostic acumen and authoritative management?

By experience, of course. But also through the knowledge accumulated by those who have faced the situation before and made important contributions by indicating the essential features to enquire about in the history, the signs to seek in the clinical examination, the laboratory measurements to order, and the first steps to take in management.

Emergencies are situations more than any others where one feels the drawbacks of our learning being divided into medical and surgical subjects, and further subdivided now into the organ specialties. House officers have to assemble in a trice knowledge from many sources. In a way, this is the strength of the young pre-registration or post-registration house officer: in this era of fast expanding knowledge he or she is, across the board, most up to date. But it demands a superb memory and a flexibility of thought given to very few of us.

Richard Robinson and Robin Stott realised the need for a pocket manual about the essentials of the current diagnostic, therapeutic and management principles, to deal properly with medical emergencies. So they have written this book, to bring together information widely scattered in textbooks on many subjects. They have set things down on the assumption, correct I believe, that the users will be the graduates of the present era, au fait with current hospital facilities and modern drugs. They have aimed to help them by concise writing. Here and there, the approach may be regarded as didactic, but that hardly matters in the emergency situation. I therefore commend this book to all those young people into whose hands our most seriously ill emergencies first come, with my best wishes to them for quick and accurate diagnosis, and to their patients, for speedy recovery!

W. J. H. Butterfield, OBE, DM, FRCP
Regis Professor of Physic, Addenbrooke's Hospital, Cambridge

Preface

The aim of this book is still to supply a framework of knowledge into which the house physician can fit his experience. Some of the facilities mentioned are not available in many hospitals. If, by creating awareness of deficiencies, patient care is improved, this book will be justified.

Since this book was first written we have become acutely aware of another dimension of its subject. The sobering fact is that the bulk of medical emergencies, which attract so much glamour and therefore money, talent and facilities, are preventable. This applies to each of the big four—coronary artery disease, cerebrovascular accidents, acute respiratory failure and overdoses. A moment's thought will show that the causes of each of these lie in the way we respond to our social and economic situation. The increasingly complex technology of medicine has been associated with the increasing isolation of its practitioners. This has led to a pre-empting by doctors of major areas of the patient's involvement with his disease. It is all too easy to treat patients in a life-threatening situation as a physiological preparation, and to overlook the fact that the patient and his family have lived with the roots of his disease, will probably continue to do so, and will have to live with its results.

Effective prevention of these conditions will probably only begin when the responsibility for health care is taken where it belongs—in the community. The effect of this aspect of treatment—which we have almost wholly ignored—will be far greater than the results obtained by the successful management of acute emergencies.

Introduction to the fifth edition

When this book was first written, 16 years ago, it was directed at the recently qualified house physician. It was designed to help him or her cope with acutely sick patients during the first few hours of their illness. The diagnostic facilities needed involved relatively simple laboratory and radiological techniques; as such they were widely available. As the house physicians' clinical experience rapidly developed, they would find themselves working more frequently without their registrar or consultant. They worked largely in a setting of casualty departments and acute medical wards.

The situation since then has been transformed. At that time medical intensive care units were rare. They have since become widespread. With them have developed improved standards of care of many of the conditions described in this book. These depend upon, amongst other things, continuous measurement of a number of cardiorespiratory variables as well as ready availability of a variety of non-invasive imaging techniques. The newly qualified house physician may well feel initially at sea in this complex scene, partly because his or her lack of experience is now in sharp contrast to the trained intensive care nurse.

A tribute to this relatively new breed of professional is long overdue from us. Without them the development of improved management in this area of medicine would not have been possible. As a result of their constant presence by the bedside, the physical and emotional pressures fall most heavily on their shoulders. Also in consequence of this, their clinical skills become finely honed. It is frequently *their* initial observations which prompt reassessment and alteration to management. They have a role in the informal training of the newly qualified doctor. In this there is nothing new. Many of us learned our initial prescribing skills from the ward sisters of our first wards, for example. Like all partnerships, it relies on mutual tact and appreciation of the other's contribution. Suffice to say, we ourselves depend increasingly heavily on, and continue to learn much from, them.

It so happens that we both have had the privilege of working in third world countries, to which copies of this book have (independently) found their way. For this reason and because we increasingly see conditions in travellers to the UK, we have included sections on problems more frequently encountered abroad.

CARDIOVASCULAR

Cardiac arrest[8,10]

Before you ever have to deal with a cardiac arrest be prepared by:

(1) knowing how to use the defibrillator,
(2) knowing how to inflate the patient with 100% oxygen.

DIAGNOSIS

Cardiac arrest can be considered to have occurred if the carotid or femoral pulses are absent. Do not waste time trying to hear the heart. There are three main mechanisms for cardiac arrest.[4]

(1) Ventricular fibrillation (approx. 80%).
(2) Asystole (approx. 15%).
(3) Electromechanical dissociation, where near-normal complexes on the ECG are not associated with an output.

However, initial management does not depend on an accurate diagnosis of the cause.

MANAGEMENT

Your aim is to reperfuse both brain and heart by undertaking closed cardiopulmonary resuscitation. If this is started immediately, and carried out efficiently, you will be able to achieve cerebral blood flows greater than 20% of normal—the minimum needed to ensure full neurological recovery. Delay exponentially reduces your chances of achieving this goal.[9] Therefore, follow the procedure outlined below.

(1) Check the time.
(2) Ensure the patient is on a firm surface and start cardiac massage at about 60 compressions per minute. Effective cardiac massage produces a femoral pulse. The forward blood flow is as much dependent on swings in intrathoracic pressure (chest pump mechanism) as direct heart compression (heart pump mechanism).

(3) Get someone to give mouth-to-mouth respiration (the aesthetics of this can be improved by laying a handkerchief over the face of the patient). It is essential to tilt the head backwards and displace the mandible forwards to maintain a patent airway while giving mouth-to-mouth respiration. Give 3–5 compressions to 1 inflation. It is neither necessary nor desirable to stop compressing the heart while your assistant inflates the chest.[5]

(4) Check that the anaesthetist and emergency trolley, ECG, or oscilloscope, and defibrillator have all been sent for.

(5) Get the bed out of the way—you will need space.

(6) Get a sucker. The patient will soon vomit if he has not already done so.

(7) Get a drip set up. Use the needle you are most familiar with. A number 1 needle taped to the skin will do. Try the antecubital fossae first. Failing this, subclavian or internal jugular puncture gives rapid reliable access to the circulation. If you are not familiar with these techniques, expose the long saphenous vein at the ankle, and under direct vision insert the needle. Do not waste time doing a formal cut down.

(8) Get a drip stand—or hang the bottle from the hooks in the curtain rail.

(9) Attach a giving set to a bottle of 8.4% bicarbonate. A nurse should do (6), (8) and (9) while you are doing (7).

(10) Run in 100 ml of 8.4% bicarbonate (i.e. 100 mmol of bicarbonate). Thereafter run in 60 ml every 15 min. Be careful; there is a tendency to give too much bicarbonate during an arrest.

(11) If the anaesthetist is not forthcoming, insert the cuffed endotracheal tube yourself—size 9 or 10 for an average-sized adult. Re-acquaint yourself with this technique by practising after each unsuccessful cardiac arrest. The patient must not become hypoxic. If you have difficulty at first, stop every 15 seconds (s) and re-inflate as in (3).

(12) Check that the tube is in the trachea by pressing the chest (and getting a puff back up the tube) or by blowing down the tube (and listening to the chest). Anchor it to the face by taping or strapping.

(13) Attach the patient to your source of oxygen supply and inflate once every 5 s—between every third or fourth chest compression.

(14) Deliver a 200 joule (J) shock with the defibrillator as soon as it arrives. If the cardiac activity is ventricular fibrillation (VF), this may be life saving. Delay—in order to establish the nature

of the cardiac arrhythmia—lessens the chances of successfully provoking a return to sinus rhythm. Delivering a shock will do the patient no harm if the heart is in asystole.[3]

Points to remember are as follows.

(i) Straddle the electrodes across the heart—preferably one on the anterior chest wall and one on the posterior.
(ii) Do not get electrode jelly smeared across the skin between the electrodes, it will conduct current. (Caution: KY jelly does not contain electrolytes and is less efficient.)
(iii) Do not stand in puddles of blood or saline.
(iv) Ensure that the electrodes are smeared with fresh jelly at each attempt.
(v) Ensure that no one else is touching the patient or the bed.

(15) Attach the patient to an ECG or an oscilloscope as soon as possible. Machines in which the defibrillator paddles also act as ECG electrodes are now available.
(16) If ventricular fibrillation persists after three or four attempts at DC conversion:

(i) Give one or both of the following drugs i.v.:

(a) Lignocaine 50 mg if VF is coarse or paroxysmal. (Lignocaine should not be used if VF is of low amplitude.)
(b) Disopyramide 100 mg.

(ii) Now try and defibrillate again.
(iii) If, after several attempts, you are still unsuccessful, one or more of the following drugs is worth trying i.v.

(a) Phenytoin sodium 100 mg.
(b) Magnesium sulphate 5–10 mmol of a 20% solution (6–12 ml).
(c) Bretylium tosylate 5 mg/kg i.v. (followed by 100 mg i.m. hourly to a maximum of 2.0 g).

Should you successfully control VF, maintain a lignocaine infusion 2–4 mg/min for 24 h.

Bad prognostic signs are:

(i) steadily decreasing amplitude of fibrillation—the amplitude may be increased by giving calcium and adrenaline;

   (ii)   a tendency for DC shock to cause asystole.

(17) If the heart is in asystole, try to restart a normal rhythm or at least provoke VF.

   (i)   Give:
         (a) atropine 1.2 mg i.v.: this relieves the cholinergic depression of the sinus and AV nodes; its use is associated with increased survival from asystolic arrest;[2]
         (b) 10 ml of 1 : 10 000 adrenaline (or 1 ml of 1 : 1000 adrenaline) i.v.;
         (c) 10 ml of 10% calcium gluconate i.v.;

   (ii)   Wait for the heart to fibrillate and then defibrillate.
   (iii) If fibrillation does not occur within 5 min, repeat the dose of adrenaline.
   (iv)   If this is not successful, give an intracardiac injection of 5 ml of 1 : 10 000 adrenaline together with 5 ml of 10% calcium gluconate. Put a chest aspiration needle on your syringe and insert this in the 4th intercostal space, to the left of the midline. Push the needle in on suction until you withdraw blood. This should be from the heart, and you can then inject the adrenaline directly into the chamber.[7]
   (v)   Continue cardiac massage to pump the injection into the coronary arteries.

(18) If the heart is in atrial asystole with widely spread ineffectual ventricular beats, provoke VF and defibrillate as above.

(19) While (13) to (17) are going on, 10–15 min will have elapsed. By this time the patient should be reasonably pink. If he is not, consider the following.

   (i)   Efforts at ventilation are insufficient. The usual tendency is to underestimate the rate and depth of ventilation needed and it is sometimes salutory to measure the blood gases during a cardiac arrest.
   (ii)   The patient has inhaled masses of vomit. Suck this out through the endotracheal tube. If your resuscitation is subsequently successful, remember to give high doses of corticosteroids as prophylaxis to vomit-induced 'shock lung' (see p. 91).
   (iii) The endotracheal tube is past the carina and is in one main bronchus. Withdraw the tube slightly. Both (iii) and

(vi) will give poor breath sounds with diminished movement on one side. If in doubt, try (iii) first.

(iv) The patient has had a massive pulmonary embolus. The lungs will resist inflation.

(v) The oxygen supply has run out. You do not know when this occurred so carry on.

(vi) The patient has a pneumothorax (see p. 80).

(20) Other points to bear in mind are:

(i) The cause of the arrest: acute hypoxia, fits, upper airway obstruction, electrolyte disturbances such as hypo- or hyperkalaemia, and digoxin poisoning are potentially reversible. Severe brain injury, massive pulmonary emboli and ruptured aortic aneurysms are not.

(ii) Full recovery has been recorded after the pupils have been fully dilated. This sign is not in itself a sufficient reason for stopping.

(iii) Do not forget cardiac tamponade (see p. 60). If due to a tense effusion, it may be necessary to aspirate the pericardial space, or if due to blood clot, an emergency thoracotomy (at the bedside) is indicated. The heart may then be defibrillated directly using internal paddles. A thoracotomy may also have to be performed if you are not obtaining an adequate circulation for some other reason, e.g. regurgitant heart valves.

(iv) Finally—and more rapidly acquired with experience than you might think—try to keep a detached attitude. When the situation is under control, e.g. the drip is up, the patient is being inflated and the ECG or oscilloscope is running, get someone else to do the cardiac massage; step back and decide what you are going to do next and for how long you are going to continue.

(21) There is increasing interest in measures which might help reduce the effects of cerebral ischaemia which occur as a consequence of the reduced cerebral circulation during cardiopulmonary resuscitation. Intracarotid injection of dextran 40 may improve cerebral outcome, and there is preliminary evidence that calcium-channel blockers may help. Other measures used to reduce intracranial pressure (see p. 205) have also been tried, without obvious benefit.[1] We, in common with others, do not think these therapies are justified at present.[6,10]

(22) Although open-heart massage has become unfashionable, it is important to remember that it is a much more efficient way of generating blood flow than is closed massage.[9] The situations where this is the process of choice are indicated below.

    (i)   Where treatable intrathoracic pathology has caused the cardiac arrest, e.g. uncontrolled haemorrhage.

    (ii)   When you cannot produce a carotid pulse by sternal compression.

    (iii) As a last step in treating intractable VF. This may particularly occur in hypothermia (see p. 265).

Technique

    (i)   Cut through skin and muscle overlying the 4th or 5th intercostal space. Pierce other intercostal structures with a blunt instrument, and spread open the intercostal space with your fingers or a rib spreader.

    (ii)   Compress the heart by placing your right hand behind it, with the thenar eminence and a thumb in front of it.

    (iii) All drugs, except for HCO_3, may safely be given via the intracardiac route.

    (iv) Defibrillation. Use insulated paddle electrodes with saline-soaked paddles. Place one behind the left ventricle, the other in front of the heart. Use 0.5 J/kg body weight initially, increasing the energy as necessary.

REFERENCES

1   Aitkenhead A. (1986). Cerebral protection. *Br. J. Hosp. Med.*; **35:** 290.

2   Camm A. J. (1986). Asystole and electromechanical dissociation. *Br. Med. J.*; **292:** 1123.

3   Campbell N. P., Webb S. W., Adgey A. A. *et al.* (1977). Transthoracic ventricular defibrillation in adults. *Br. Med. J.*, **2:** 1379.

4   Chamberlain D. (1986). Ventricular fibrillation. *Br. Med. J.*; **292:** 1068.

5   Chandras N., Rudiboff M., Weisfeldt M. I. (1980). Simultaneous chest compression and ventilation at high airway pressure during cardiopulmonary resuscitation. *Lancet*; **i:** 175.

6   Dearden N. M. (1985). Ischaemic brain. *Lancet*; **ii:** 255.

7   Sabun H. I. *et al.* (1983). Accuracy of intracardiac injections determined by post-mortem study. *Lancet*; **ii:** 1054.
8   Safar P. (1981). *Cardiopulmonary Cerebral Resuscitation.* Philadelphia: W. B. Saunders.
9   Safar P. (1984). Recent advances in cardiopulmonary–cerebral resuscitation: a review. *Ann. Emer. Med.*; **13:** 856.
10   Yatsu F. M. (1986). Cardiopulmonary–cerebral resuscitation. *N. Engl. J. Med.*; **314**: 446.

Myocardial infarction

DIAGNOSIS

(1) Myocardial infarction usually presents with a history of severe crushing retrosternal chest pain, often radiating to the neck and arms. The patient often perspires and is nauseated. Those with previous angina fail to obtain the usual relief from nitrates.

(2) However, it may present in a number of indirect ways, particularly in the elderly, for example:

(i)   acute left ventricular failure,
(ii)   unexplained hypotension (commonly postoperative),
(iii)   a peripheral embolus,
(iv)   fainting, giddy turns, palpitations or 'collapse',
(v)   a stroke—either due to (ii) or (iii),
(vi)   diabetic ketoacidosis.

Remember that the pain may be felt in the traditional referral sites only.

(3) It is sometimes difficult to be sure that a myocardial infarction has occurred.[11] In such cases, the patient must be admitted for observation, and serial ECGs and cardiac enzyme studies undertaken. The creatine phosphokinase (CPK) is particularly useful, as it invariably rises within the 12 hours (h) after infarction. A rise in CPK due to other causes, e.g. intramuscular injections, may be distinguished by assaying the MB CPK isoenzyme which is more prevalent in cardiac muscle. A normal ECG does not exclude the diagnosis of myocardial infarction, as it may have been recorded too early. A proportion of these patients may have the preinfarction syndrome (see p. 21).

MANAGEMENT

All patients must have either a drip or a heparinised cannula (Venflon) inserted. Drugs must be given i.v., both for speed and because absorption by other routes is uncertain when perfusion is diminished. Then three factors, given below in order of priority, need urgent attention.

(1) Pain control.

(i) Diamorphine 5 mg i.v. and morphine 10–15 mg i.v. (each with 50 mg cyclizine or 12.5 mg prochlorperazine 1 min beforehand to forestall vomiting) are still the drugs of choice. The new synthetic narcotic agents have no advantage over these two drugs. Pentazocine (Fortral) may cause a rise in pulmonary artery pressure and should not be used.

(ii) Isosorbide dinitrate, given in a starting dose of 2–10 mg/h i.v., may be used to relieve pain which is unrelieved by heroin within 6–12 h. Until the i.v. infusion is underway, give sublingual glyceryl trinitrate 0.5 mg ¼-hourly. In addition to its role in pain relief, there may be other reasons for giving nitrates (see p. 42).

(iii) Under no circumstances withhold these drugs from patients suffering from myocardial pain. If you are worried about the possibility of respiratory depression, monitor the blood gases and treat appropriately (q.v.) However, if necessary, respiratory and circulatory depression due to narcotics can be counteracted by:

(a) naloxone 0.4–1.2 mg i.v. in divided doses over 3 min,
(b) nalorphine 5–10 mg repeated to a dose of 40 mg, if you do not have naloxone,
(c) doxapram, by continuous infusion, 1.5 mg/min to a maximum of 2.5 mg/min.

(2) Arrhythmias must be treated (see p. 23). Bradycardia in the acute stage should be treated with atropine 0.6–2.4 mg i.v.[22]

(3) Heart failure.

(i) This may be due to (1) or (2) above, which should be treated appropriately. Otherwise impaired ventricular function results, either from loss of functioning muscle or from mechanical disruption of the ventricular wall (VSD or rupture of the wall with tamponade) or valves (acute mitral regurgitation). Mechanical disruption usually occurs later in the course of the disease (2–10 days).

(ii) Invasive haemodynamic studies in normal subjects show that cardiac output is between 2.2 and 4.3 litres/m² per min. If measured cardiac output falls below 2.2 litres/m² per min, clinical symptoms of poor perfusion (cool peripheries, hypotension, oliguria and a tendency toward mental confusion) appear. This is called pump failure. Similarly, normal pulmonary capillary wedge pressure (PCWP, an indirect measure of left atrial pressure) is below 18 mmHg. If the PCWP exceeds 25 mmHG, the signs of pulmonary oedema develop (see p. 39): dyspnoea, added heart sounds, late inspiratory crackles on auscultation, and enlargement of the pulmonary veins, particularly to the upper lobe, on the chest x-ray, all this with or without radiological oedema. Heart failure and left ventricular failure are therefore unhelpful terms since they may refer either to pulmonary oedema or to the consequences of low cardiac output (pump failure), or both

(iii) Haemodynamics studies in patients with myocardial infarction, measuring cardiac output and pulmonary wedge pressure, have shown that there are four groups of patients.[7]

Since the clinical picture correlates well with the haemodynamic findings (see (ii) above) we use the following clinical classification on which to build a rational approach to therapy.

Table 1

Group	Clinical features	Haemodynamic characteristics	Average mortality
a	No pulmonary oedema	Normal PCWP ($<$18 mmHg)	1%
	Good perfusion	Normal cardiac output ($>$2.2 l/min)	
b	Pulmonary oedema	Raised PCWP ($>$25 mmHg)	10%
	Good perfusion	Normal cardiac output	
c	No pulmonary oedema Poor perfusion—pump failure	Normal PCWP Low cardiac output ($<$2.2 l/min)	20%
d	Pulmonary oedema Poor perfusion—pump failure	Raised PCWP Low cardiac output	60%

TREATMENT

Group a

(1) No specific therapy is required, but therapy directed at reducing infarct size is being investigated, as it is clear that the prognosis after infarction relates to the infarct size.[2]

(2) Infarct size may, in principle, be reduced by reducing heart work, increasing perfusion, or preferably both, working on the assumption that there will be a critical period after the infarct when ischaemic zones of myocardium are recoverable.[1] This seems to be the case if effective intervention takes place within 4 h of the onset of symptoms. In view of the fact that 80% of acute infarcts are consequent to thrombosis in the coronary vessels,[5] any substantial increase in perfusion really means clot lysis, bypass surgery or coronary angioplasty.[8] These last two require specialised skills unlikely to be available in district hospitals, so the available options are as follows.

(i) Vasodilators, such as the nitrates. The main effect of these is venodilatation, with a reduction in preload and, to a lesser extent, arteriolar dilatation, with a reduction in afterload. Both these will reduce heart work.[6] Some direct dilatation of the coronary vessels may also occur. The consensus is that these may have some beneficial effect in reducing infarct size, but until the situation is clearer, we do not think that they should be routinely used for this purpose.

(ii) β-Blockers.[14] Whether these agents reduce infarct size by reducing both heart rate and arterial pressure, and therefore heart work, is not certain. The most promising results have been obtained with i.v. timolol. The initial dose is 1 mg i.v., followed 10 min later by a further 1 mg, and then 10 min later by a continual infusion of 0.6 mg/h for 24 h. Thereafter, 10 mg b.d. is given orally.[5] We do not use this therapy as a routine. Clearly nobody with contra-indications to β-blockers—A–V dissociation, pulmonary oedema, hypotension (systolic BP <100 mmHg) bradycardia (pulse rate <60/min) or concurrent administration of any other antiarrhythmic agent—should be given this therapy.

(iii) Thrombolytic therapy.[8,12,17] Streptokinase has been given directly into coronary arteries, with lysis of clot in about 75% of cases. This method is impractical for general use, but i.v. streptokinase in a dose of around 1 000 000 units over 1 h is effective in lysing clot in around 50% of patients. However, we believe that the routine use of thrombolytics should await the general availability of tissue-type plasminogen activators. Initial studies with the i.v. use of these is promising in that 80% recanalisation rates are achieved.[20]

Group b

(1) A diuretic such as frusemide 20–40 mg i.v. is the best means of reducing pulmonary wedge pressure and relieving pulmonary congestion.

(2) You should monitor the dose in accordance with your patient's response. Clinical improvement often precedes both radiological improvement and the disappearance of physical signs. An excessive diuresis can cause hypovolaemia, so bear this lag phenomenon in mind when adjusting diuretic doses. Conversely, tachypnoea, as a result of decreased lung compliance, will precede the development of frank pulmonary oedema.

(3) Digoxin. Do not use this routinely. In a situation of deteriorating failure, the therapy outlined under 'group d' should be used.

Groups c and d

These two constitute the entity previously called 'cardiogenic shock'. Before embarking on therapy it is invaluable to have a Swan–Ganz catheter in place to measure PCWP; ideally cardiac output should also be measured, as should central venous pressure (CVP), but it is only an indirect, and hence frequently misleading, indication of left ventricular function. However, changes in CVP taken in conjunction with clinical observations can provide a basis on which to act (see p. 342).

Group c

It is mandatory to exclude hypovolaemia in this group, and this is most conveniently done by measuring the PCWP which will be low in hypovolaemia. Hypovolaemia after infarction is more common than generally appreciated, and may be explained in some (though not all) patients by the prolonged periods of anorexia, vomiting or sweating that accompany infarction. Therefore, proceed as follows.

(1) Give i.v. Haemaccel or dextran 70 made in 5% dextrose, or plasma, or albumin, until the PCWP approaches 18 mmHg or until the CVP approaches the upper normal range without the development of tachypnoea.

(2) If hypovolaemia has been treated or excluded, pump failure may be a consequence of an inadequate heart rate in the presence of a low fixed stroke volume. Treat sinus bradycardia with atropine and heart block or slow atrial fibrillation with a pacemaker set at 90–100 beats/min. Remember that atrial transport may contribute up to 30% of cardiac output so that pacing of a refractory sinus bradycardia may achieve little improvement in output. It is better to use isoprenaline or dopamine (see below).

(3) For persistent pump failure with an adequate rate and volume, proceed as for group d.

Group d

(1) Many of these patients will die, but treatment may occasionally be gratifyingly successful. Rational treatment is based on the idea that the ischaemic myocardium will function best given an optimal supply of oxygen and a minimum amount of work to do. We cannot often improve oxygen supply, so the above aim is best achieved using vasodilators. These come in two guises:

(i) venodilators, which act primarily to reduce the PCWP and thus the preload on the left ventricle;

(ii) arteriodilators, which reduce peripheral resistance, and thus the afterload on the left ventricle.

(2) Therefore use the following.

(i) Sodium nitroprusside 0.5–10 μg/kg per min.[10] Nitroprusside, which, because it has a roughly equal effect on veins and arteries is called a balanced vasodilator, has a half-life of 2–5 min. It may cause profound hypotension[18] (though, paradoxically, this is less likely to happen with patients who are more ill). Careful titration of the dose using intra-arterial monitoring is therefore mandatory. We use a short cannula—usually an 18-gauge Venflon in the radial artery. Electronic monitoring is ideal, but an anaeroid (Tychos) gauge or even direct manometry using a manometer line strung up on a tall drip stand may be satisfactory. If you cannot use nitroprusside for lack of intra-arterial monitoring, use salbutamol.

(ii) Salbutamol, 3–20 μg/min. This acts primarily as a vaso-dilator and may be managed using routine reading of CVP and BP.

(3) The persistence of unacceptably poor perfusion is indicated by:

(i) an hourly urine output of less than 0.5 ml/kg per h,

(ii) a core peripheral (rectal/toe) temperature gap of >5°C.

(4) In these circumstances there is little alternative but to resort to inotropic agents, with the possible dangers of increasing the oxygen demand of the myocardium more than supply to it. The choices are as follows.

(i) Dopamine and/or dobutamine 2–5 μg/kg per min.[9] In this dose range dopamine has little overall effect on systemic resistance; however, the preferential increase in renal flow makes it the catecholamine of choice. If a dopamine infusion of 5 μg/kg per min has not restored perfusion, it is wise to add dobutamine, starting at a dose of 2.5 μg/kg per min, and increasing to 10 μg/kg per min as necessary. Dobutamine is a more potent inotrope than dopamine, but does not have the renal vasodilator effect. Thus using the two together optimises the benefits of both, and also makes good pharmacological sense.

(ii) If neither of these is available, use isoprenaline, 0.5–10 μg/min.

(5) Digitalisation is a form of inotropic support which seems to have little theoretical advantage over the catecholamines. However, some clinicians feel unhappy if their patients are not digitalised in these circumstances, in which case a quick-acting compound with a short half-life seems preferable. We use ouabain, which acts within 5–10 min, has its peak effect within 0.5–2 h, and which has a half-life of 21 h (digoxin's half-life is 36 h). The starting dose of ouabain is 500 μg i.v., repeated at 4-hourly intervals as necessary, to a maximum of 2.0 mg in 24 h. Digoxin itself is a perfectly satisfactory alternative; give an initial dose of 1.0 mg i.v., and then 0.5 mg 6-hourly to a maximum of 2.5 mg.

(6) Infuse 500 ml of 20% glucose, containing 39 mmol KCl and 20 units of soluble insulin (GIK) over 6 h. This is said to improve myocardial contractility, but its use is controversial. This same regimen may also be helpful in the 'sick cell syndrome'. Here the sodium pump, which is responsible for the extrusion of sodium from cells, falters. The intracellular sodium rises as the extracellular sodium falls, and the altered ionic millieu causes widespread, and often disastrous, metabolic consequences. The sick cell syndrome often occurs as a terminal event in many serious illnesses, and so the above regimen is only occasionally helpful.

(7) Balloon pumping is theoretically the most potent intervention in these circumstances.[10] If balloon pumping is available, it must be used early; it is unlikely to be of any value in patients who have had the signs of pump failure for longer than 4 h. It is of particular value when combined with surgery in the management of mechanical disruption of the ventricle.

Having put in a venous line and treated pain, arrhythmias and failure, consider the following.

(1) Anxiety. Many patients are already aware of their diagnosis, and it provides for them a most potent intimation of mortality. Reassurance is of paramount importance, if necessary supported by diazepam 5–10 mg i.v. or 2–5 mg t.d.s. orally. Lorazepam 1–4 mg i.v. or 1–2 mg t.d.s. orally is another excellent sedative.

(2) Give oxygen (40%) via an MC mask as even patients with minor infarcts may have a low Pao_2.

(3) Anticoagulants.[3,16,21] Heparin 5000 units subcutaneously 8-hourly, started within 8 h of the infarction, prevents thromboembolism as effectively as conventional full anticoagulation. In addition, hypertension and peptic ulceration are not contraindications to this regimen. Full anticoagulation should probably be used in patients with a full thickness anterior infarct, as this group is particularly prone to forming intraventricular clots. To achieve this, i.v. heparin may be given either intermittently 10 000 units 6-hourly, or, preferably, by continuous infusion using a suitable pump. In this case start with 10 000 units 6-hourly, but monitor the dose to keep the partial thromboplastin time (PTT) between two and four times normal.

With either of the above regimens, we suggest continuing heparin for 5 days. In the evening of the last 3 days give warfarin 9 mg orally. On the sixth day, switch to warfarin exclusively, with the dosage monitored by the prothrombin time. Remember that heparin is inactivated by dextrose; only infuse it in normal saline.

(4) Streptokinase. The use of this in early infarction is discussed on p. 13.

(5) Check the blood sugar. Many patients with an infarct develop stress-induced hyperglycaemia, and raised sugar may predispose towards arrhythmias.[4] Persistent hyperglycaemia should be treated in the acute situation with an i.v. insulin infusion (see p. 153), commencing at a dose of 2 units/h. Subsequent doses should be given as indicated below.

Blood glucose (mmol/l)	<4	4–8	8–12	12–22	22+
Insulin (units/h)	0	0.5	1	2	4

There is some evidence that careful control of the blood sugar after infarction improves the prognosis, probably by reducing the incidence of cardiac arrhythmias.[4]

(6) Pericarditis. Pericarditis and minor pericardial effusions are common after a myocardial infarct.

　　(i)　Pericardial pain is quickly relieved with a non-steroidal anti-inflammatory drug (NSAID).

　　(ii)　The presence of pericarditis should not influence your decision about anticoagulants. Contrary to what you might expect, these can be safely used in patients with pericarditis.[13]

(7) Routine lignocaine prophylaxis.[15] The concept of warning arrhythmias has proven to be unhelpful, and ventricular fibrillation occurs both with and without warning after myocardial infarction. The incidence decreases exponentially with time, and, as a primary electrical problem, is rare after 24 h. Some would therefore advocate routine lignocaine prophylaxis after all infarcts. However, as the detection and correction of ventricular fibrillation in our coronary care unit are so good, and lignocaine is potentially toxic, we reserve its use for those who have had an episode of ventricular fibrillation. In this group, give a bolus of 100 mg i.v. and then give a continuous infusion at 4 mg/min for 1 h. Reduce the dose to 2.0 mg/min, and then

stop the infusion after 24 h. In people over the age of 65, or with hepatic dysfunction, reduce the above dose by one-third.
(8) Magnesium. Recent evidence suggests that 50 mmol of magnesium (as $MgCl_2$) infused in 1000 ml of isotonic glucose over the 24 h after admission, and a further 16 mmol in the next 24 h, reduces the mortality of patients with an acute myocardial infarction. This therapy has the virtue of being harmless and seems to us to be well worth trying.[19]

REFERENCES

General

Bradley R. A. (1977). *Studies in Acute Heart Failure*. London. Edward Arnold.
Hillis L. D., Braunwald E. (1977). Myocardial ischaemia. *N. Engl. J. Med.*; **296:** 971.

Specific

1 Breckenbridge A. (1982). Vasodilators in heart failure. *Br. Med. J.*; **284:** 763.
2 Bulkeley B. (1981). Site and sequelae of myocardial infarction. *N. Engl. J. Med.*; **305:** 337.
3 Chalmers R. J., Smith H. Jr, Kunzler A. M. (1977). Evidence favouring the use of anticoagulants in the hospital phase of acute myocardial infarction. *N. Engl. J. Med.*; **297:** 1091.
4 Clark R., English M. (1985). Effects of intravenous infusion of insulin in diabetics with acute myocardial infarction. *Br. Med. J.*; **291:** 303.
5 Collaborative Study (1984). Reduction in infarct size with the early use of timolol in acute myocardial infarction. *N. Engl. J. Med.*; **310:** 9.
6 DeWood M. A. *et al.* (1980). Prevalence of total coronary occlusion during the early hours of transmural infarction. *N. Engl. J. Med.*; **303:** 897.
7 Forrester J. S., Diamond G., Chaterjee K. *et al.* (1976/1977). Medical therapy of acute myocardial infarction by application of haemodynamic subsets. *N. Engl. J. Med.*; **295:** 1356, **296:** 971, 1034, 1093.
8 Laffel G. L., Braunwald E. (1984). Thrombolytic therapy. *N. Engl. J. Med.*; **311:** 710.
9 Leader (1977). Intravenous dopamine. *Lancet*; **ii:** 231.

10   Leader (1980). The intra-aortic balloon pump. *Br. Med. J.*;
      281: 764.
11   Leader (1982). Diagnosis of doubtful coronary. *Lancet*; **i:** 661.
12   Leader (1986). Streptokinase in acute myocardial infarct.
      Lancet; **i:** 421.
13   Leader (1986). Pericardial effusion after acute myocardial
      infarction. *Lancet*; **i:** 1015.
14   Leader (1986). Intravenous β-blockade during acute myocar-
      dial infarction. *Lancet*; **ii:** 79.
15   Lown B. (1985). Lignocaine to prevent ventricular
      fibrillation—easy does it. *N. Engl. J. Med.*; **313:** 1154.
16   Mitchell J. R. A. (1981). Anticoagulants in coronary heart
      disease—retrospect and prospect. *Lancet*; **i:** 257.
17   Mitchell J. R. A. (1986). Back to the future: so what will
      fibrinolytic therapy offer your patients with myocardial infarc-
      tion? *Br. Med. J.*; **292:** 973.
18   Passamani E. R. (1982). Nitroprusside in myocardial infarc-
      tion. *N. Engl. J. Med.*; **306:** 1168.
19   Rasmussen H. *et al.* (1986). Intravenous magnesium in acute
      myocardial infarct. *Lancet*; **i:** 234.
20   Relman A. S. (1985). Intravenous thrombolysis in acute
      myocardial infarction. *N. Engl. J. Med.*; **312:** 915.
21   Warlow C., Terry G., Kenmore A. C. *et al.* (1973). Double
      blind trial of low doses of subcutaneous heparin in the preven-
      tion of deep vein thrombosis after myocardial infarction.
      Lancet; **ii:** 934.
22   Webb S. W., Adgey A. A., Pantridge J. F. (1972). Autonomic
      disturbance at onset of acute myocardial infarction. *Br. Med.
      J.*; **3:** 89.

Preinfarction syndrome (unstable angina)[1,2,4,5]

DIAGNOSIS

The preinfarction syndrome consists of the following.

(1) Recurrent angina at rest.
(2) Increasing angina not rapidly relieved by glyceryl trinitrate.
(3) Variable and transient ECG changes.
(4) Normal enzyme levels.

It is that part of the spectrum of ischaemic heart disease which lies between stable effort angina and a myocardial infarction. We sometimes have difficulty in knowing at which precise point in the spectrum an individual patient is; when there is this dilemma, for therapeutic reasons it is best to err on the side of a diagnosis of unstable angina rather than an infarct.

About one in seven of these patients will progress to myocardial infarction in the short term if left untreated. Recent evidence suggests that the dominant cause of both the initial symptoms and the progression to a full-blown infarct is a reduction in coronary blood flow rather than an increase in myocardial oxygen consumption. Therefore the main therapeutic endeavour is directed toward improving flow. In effect this means using vasodilators and drugs which, by reducing platelet aggregation, reduce the tendency to form intracoronary thrombi.

MANAGEMENT

(1) Anxiety and pain should be managed as for myocardial infarction.
(2) Nitrates. Until you have established an i.v. infusion (see below), give glyceryl trinitrate 0.5 mg sublingually ¼-hourly. Start i.v. isosorbide dinitrate as soon as possible, initially at 2 mg/h. This can be increased to a maximum of 10 mg/h. You should aim for the lowest dose which will achieve pain relief whilst not reducing the systolic arterial pressure (which is best monitored with an arterial line) below 100 mmHg. After your patient has been pain free for 6 h, start oral nitrates (e.g.

isosorbide mononitrate 20–40 mg twice daily), and tail off the i.v. infusion.

(3) Give propranolol in a dose sufficient either to stop pain or to reduce the pulse rate below 50 beats/min. Start at 20 mg 4-hourly (orally) and increase as necessary. The original rationale for using β-blockers was to reduce myocardial oxygen consumption. However, as has been suggested above, this does not appear to be the main cause of the problem, and it may be that the antiplatelet aggregation effect of propranolol is the important one.[5] Atenolol 50 mg b.d. is a suitable alternative β-blocker.

(4) If, despite the above measures, the pain persists for 24 h, add nifedipine 10–20 mg three times a day.[6]

(5) Formal anticoagulation with heparin may not prevent the development of infarction but is indicated on the same basis as in myocardial infarction. Aspirin, in a dose of 325 mg/day, has been shown to be beneficial in one large trial, presumably due to its antiplatelet effect.[3] We now use it routinely.

(6) Patients whose symptoms persist for 48 h despite the above therapy, and in whom there is no evidence of infarction, should be considered for coronary arteriography with a view to surgery. Intra-aortic balloon pump assistance before surgery should be considered.

(7) Fibrinolytics. The use of these agents in the preinfarction syndrome is on the same basis as in early myocardial infarction (see p. 13). We anticipate that any benefit will be greater in preinfarction.

(8) Coronary angioplasty.[1] The situation here is as for fibrinolytics.

REFERENCES

1   De Feyter P. J. *et al.* (1985). Emergency coronary angioplasty in refractory unstable angina. *N. Engl. J. Med.*; **313:** 342.

2   Leader (1982). Unstable angina. *Lancet*; **ii:** 569.

3   Lewis H. D. *et al.* (1983). Protective effects of aspirin against acute myocardial infarction and death in men with unstable angina. *N. Engl. J. Med.*; **309:** 396.

4   Maseri A. (1983). The changing face of angina pectoris—practical implications. *Lancet;* **i:** 746.

5   Oliva P. B. (1984). Unstable rest angina with ST segment depression. *Ann. Intern Med.*; **100:** 424.

6   Zelis R. (1982). Calcium blocker therapy for unstable angina pectoris. *N. Engl. J. Med.*; **306:** 926.

Cardiac arrhythmias

These may be supraventricular, arising from the atria (atrial) or from around the A-V node (junctional), or ventricular, arising below the A-V node. They cause too rapid a heart action (tachycardia), occasional irregularities in rhythm (extrasystoles) or too slow a heart action (bradycardia). Also included in this section are arrhythmias due to an abnormal relationship between atrial and ventricular contraction (conduction defects).

Arrhythmias are encountered commonly after myocardial infarction. They may occur terminally after a period of hypotension and congestive cardiac failure, in which case they are usually resistant to treatment (so-called secondary arrhythmias). However, they may also occur as a temporary disturbance in a heart capable of maintaining an adequate circulation. It is in this group, the primary arrhythmias, that treatment may be life saving.

Arrhythmias may be potentiated or even caused by the following.

(1) Pain and anxiety—always ask your patient specifically about the presence of pain; he may be stoical.
(2) Hypoxia (which is often impossible to detect clinically).
(3) Acidosis.
(4) Hypo- or hyperkalaemia.
(5) Hypo- or hypercalcaemia.
(6) Hypomagnesaemia.
(7) Sick cell syndrome (the escape of Na^+ into and K^+ out of cells is potentially reversible with glucose, K^+ and insulin; see p. 13).

Correction of these abnormalities may stop the arrhythmia and will certainly make it more amenable to treatment.

Arrhythmias cause their adverse effects in one or more of the following ways.

(1) Loss of atrial transport, which may cause a 25% reduction in the cardiac output.
(2) Increase in myocardial oxygen requirement, coupled with decreased supply. Tachycardias (>100 beats/min), whilst causing a rate-dependent increase in consumption, also cause decreased perfusion because of the invariable shortening of diastole. Bradycardias (<40 beats/min), whilst lengthening diastole, diminish perfusion by reducing cardiac output.

(3) Loss of synchronous or organised ventricular contraction, leading to reduced output. Ventricular fibrillation is the most extreme form of this.

SUPRAVENTRICULAR ARRHYTHMIAS

Atrial ectopics (Fig. 1)

These may be caused by digoxin and catecholamines. They may occur in otherwise normal hearts, especially during pregnancy, and after myocardial infarction when they are usually benign, but they may occasionally herald atrial tachycardia or fibrillation. In this situation, as at other times, they are not treated other than by reassurance and, if necessary, mild sedation.

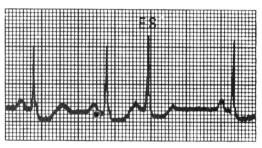

Fig. 1 Supraventricular extrasystole. The small pointed P wave can be seen deforming the preceding T wave. (ES = extrasystole.)

Supraventricular tachycardia

(1) *Sinus tachycardia* comes on gradually; its rate is affected by posture, exercise and atropine and is usually below 150 beats/min. There is always an underlying cause such as LVF, anxiety, fever or hypoxia, which should be looked for and treated as necessary. It needs to be differentiated from paroxysmal tachycardia.

(2) *Paroxysmal tachycardia* (Fig. 2) comes on abruptly. Its rate (usually >150 beats/min) is unaffected by any of the above but may be terminated by vagal stimulation. This tachycardia may be caused by digoxin, a factor which profoundly influences its treatment. If the patient is not on digoxin, the following options are available.

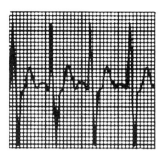

Fig. 2 Supraventricular tachycardia. The P wave can be clearly seen preceding each QRS complex.

(i) Do nothing—if there is no evidence of failure and the patient tells you that his attacks are shortlived.

(ii) Intense vagal stimulation may control this arrhythmia. Traditionally, carotid massage is used to evoke this response. The carotid sinus is level with the upper border of the thyroid cartilage. Press it firmly against the vertebral transverse process with a thumb and rub slowly 1 cm (0.5 inch) up and down the artery. Only massage one side at a time, checking first that there are no carotid bruits, whose presence constitutes a contraindication. A newer approach is to make use of the 'diving response', which can be induced clinically by placing an ice bag on the patient's face.[7]

(iii) The treatment of choice in patients whose circulation is compromised, and which is nearly always successful, is synchronised DC reversion. This is carried out with an anaesthetist who gives a short-acting anaesthetic (thiopentone 100–500 mg i.v., ketamine—a bolus of 2 mg/kg given i.v. over 60 s gives 15 min anaesthesia—or etomidate 300 mg/kg by slow i.v. injection). Ventilatory equipment should be available in case a temporary period of apnoea occurs. Give the shock observing the usual precautions (see p. 5), starting at 100 J and increasing the stimulus by 50 J increments until 400 J are reached. If this is ineffective, try placing one 'paddle' on the patient's back behind the heart and one in front. If DC reversion has been unsuccessful, you should try it again after giving one of the drugs mentioned below.

(iv) If DC reversion is either not available or not considered necessary, the following drugs may be useful.

(a) Verapamil, a depressor of A-V nodal function, 5 mg i.v. repeated at 5 min intervals to a maximum of 20 mg is usually effective. This should not be used if any other antiarrhythmic drug has been given before it, or if the patient is in shock, as it may cause irreversible asystole. It is emerging as the drug of choice in supraventricular tachycardias however.

(b) Assuming your patient is not already on digoxin, a cardiac glycoside, such as ouabain, or digoxin itself may be used (see p. 16).

(c) Try carotid sinus massage or a facial cold shock again after (a) and (b).

(d) Amiodarine 5 mg/kg infused over 20 min through a long intracath may be tried.[1] If this is successful, it may be continued as a continuous infusion, 600–1200 mg over 24 h.

(e) β-Blockers. These are still used in some places as first-line therapy. Metoprolol, given in 5 mg aliquots i.v. at 5 min intervals to a maximum of 20 mg is a reasonable choice.

(f) Drugs in (a), (b) and (d) above should be given slowly to minimise any adverse circulatory effects.

Atrial flutter (Fig. 3)

This may occur after myocardial infarction and with cardiomyopathies, ASD and systemic infections. Unlike atrial fibrillation,

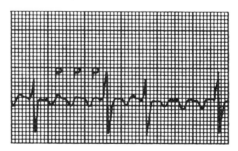

Fig. 3 Atrial flutter. The first three flutter waves are marked 'P'. The ventricles respond at a varying 1 : 2–1 : 3 ratio.

it is not associated with mitral stenosis or thyrotoxicosis. The atrium 'flutters' at an average rate of 300 beats/min. As the ventricles cannot respond at this rate, there is always some degree of 'block' which may vary (Fig. 3).

(1) The treatment of choice for the patient whose circulation is compromised is DC reversion.

(2) If this either fails or is not deemed necessary, digitalise the patient. This may cause a reversion to sinus rhythm, or progression to atrial fibrillation.

(3) Verapamil or metoprolol may be given as for atrial tachycardia. These drugs do not revert the flutter to sinus rhythm, but merely reduce the ventricular rate.

Atrial fibrillation and flutter fibrillation[1,11] (Figs. 4 and 5)

(1) For practical purposes these are the same thing.

(2) The most common cause is acute or chronic ischaemic heart disease, but it also occurs in hypertensives, in ethanolic heart disease, in association with mitral valve disease, thyrotoxicosis, subacute bacterial endocarditis, atrial septal defect, pericarditis and after thoracotomy.

(3) If the ventricular rate is sufficiently fast to cause cardiac failure, the treatment of choice is digitalisation—combined if necessary with diuretics and oxygen (see pp. 16 and 41 respectively). Continue that dose of digoxin which maintains the ventricular rate between 70 and 80 beats/min.

(4) DC reversion is unlikely to succeed if long-standing coronary artery disease is present, but should be considered electively after treatment of, for example, mitral stenosis or thyrotoxicosis (see p. 25).

(5) If digoxin is not effective, flecanide, an agent which slows intra-atrial conduction as well as producing A-V block, can be used in a dose of 2 mg/kg i.v. infusion. It is said to terminate about 70% of cases of atrial fibrillation.

(6) Remember that resistant atrial fibrillation may be a complication of pericarditis. If you are having trouble controlling it, make sure you have either excluded pericarditis or treated it with indomethacin.

Sinus bradycardia

(1) Sinus bradycardia may occur with vasovagal attacks, intracranial hypertension, myxoedema (see p. 176) and in athletes in training.

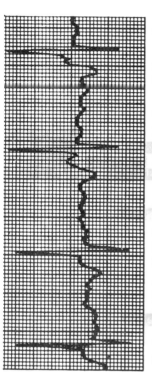

Fig. 4 Atrial flutter fibrillation. Coarse atrial activity is seen linking each QRS complex.

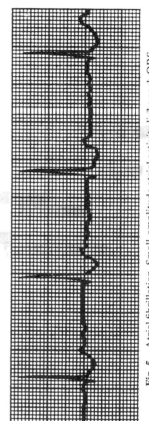

Fig. 5 Atrial fibrillation. Small-amplitude atrial activity links each QRS complex.

It is occasionally caused by β-adrenergic blocking agents, ganglion-blocking hypotensive agents (e.g. guanethidine, especially when combined with digoxin) and by digoxin itself.

(2) Bradycardia may also cause all the signs of severe cardio-vascular collapse when it occurs after inferior myocardial infarction. In this situation give atropine 0.6 mg i.v. Repeat this dose if there is no effect within 5 min. Response is usually prompt and gratifying. Atropine may cause ventricular fibrillation, urinary retention and glaucoma, and it is unwise to give more than 2.4 mg.

Isoprenaline (see p. 36) may be used if atropine fails and treatment is deemed necessary. Rarely, pacing may be necessary.

Sinus arrest[6] (Fig. 6)

Sinus arrest may be caused by many of the antiarrhythmic drugs, hyperkalaemia, autonomic instability (as in the Guillain-Barré syndrome), and myocardial infarction. Short periods of sinus inactivity may progress to permanent sinus arrest and, if they occur, a transvenous intracardiac pacemaker should be passed urgently. Prior to this, sinus rhythm may be restored by a sharp precordial blow or by atropine 0.6–2.4 mg i.v.

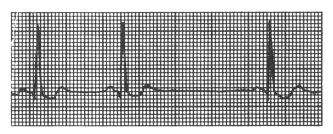

Fig. 6   Sinus arrest. After the second beat there is a temporary delay in sinus activity before the third beat is initiated.

Junctional arrhythmias (Figs. 7, 8 and 9)

Junctional rhythms represent the action of a natural pacemaker at variable sites in the bundle of His which takes over as a result of sinus node dysfunction, the commonest causes of which are digoxin toxicity, myocardial infarction and myocarditis. If the rate is sufficiently slow to cause cardiac failure, atropine 0.6–2.4 mg i.v.

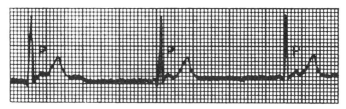

Fig. 7   Junctional rhythm. The P wave of each beat is clearly seen deforming the ST segment.

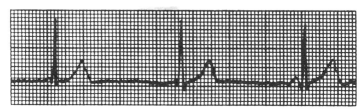

Fig. 8   Junctional rhythm. The P wave is seen immediately preceding each QRS complex.

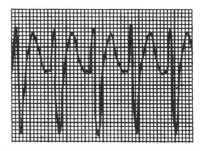

Fig. 9   Junctional tachycardia. A small P wave is seen immediately preceding each wide QRS complex.

may provoke the sinus node to return at the normal rate. Failing this, isoprenaline (see p. 36) may encourage acceleration of the junctional rhythms. Junctional tachycardias are treated as their atrial counterparts.

VENTRICULAR ARRHYTHMIAS [2]

Ventricular ectopics (Fig. 10)

(1) These occur in myocardial infarction and in cardiomyopathies or as a result of digoxin toxicity.

(2) They may herald ventricular tachycardia or fibrillation (death, although sudden, is not always unannounced) if:

    (i) they interrupt the T wave or ST segment of the preceding complex (in technical terms, if their coupling interval is short),

    (ii) they are of multifocal origin,

    (iii) they are frequent (more than 10/min),

    (iv) more than two occur in succession.

However, the relevance of these warning arrhythmias has certainly been overstated.

(3) They may be provoked by pain, hypoxia or hypokalaemia.

    (i) If treatment of these circumstances does not improve matters, give lignocaine 100 mg i.v. as a bolus followed by an infusion at 4 mg/min. Reduce the infusion dose as soon as possible, usually within 1 h, to 2 mg/min. (See p. 19 for the circumstances in which you need to alter the above dose schedule.)

    (ii) If this fails, use the following.

        (a) Disopyramide 2 mg/kg i.v. as a loading dose, and then up to 1 g/day i.v. or orally.[5]

        (b) Procainamide. Give 100 mg i.v. diluted in 5% dextrose, at a rate not exceeding 25–50 mg/min. This dose can be repeated at 5–10 min intervals until the

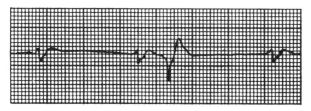

Fig. 10   Ventricular ectopic beat.

arrhythmia is controlled, adverse reactions occur, or the maximum of 1.0 g has been given. To maintain therapeutic levels, give 2–6 mg/min by continuous infusion.

(c) Amiodarone 5–10 mg/kg i.v. over 20 min, then 600–1200 mg via a continuous infusion over 24 h.

(d) Bretylium tosylate (see p. 5).

After myocardial infarction a few ventricular ectopics are very common. If they do not have the characteristics outlined in (a)–(d) above, just observe.

Ventricular tachycardia (Figs. 11 and 12)

(1) This may be difficult to distinguish from supraventricular tachycardia with bundle branch block because:

(i)   the clinical signs which frequently occur in ventricular tachycardia, namely:

(a) occasional cannon waves,
(b) varying intensity of first heart sound,

are not always present and can occur in SVT with bundle branch block; and

(ii) the ECG features commonly associated with ventricular tachycardia, namely:

(a) P waves in varying relationship to QRS complexes,
(b) slight irregularity of the QRS complex and rate,

may occur in either condition.

However, the majority of wide complex tachycardias are ventricular in origin. Distinguishing ECG features are unreliable. Treating ventricular tachycardias as supraventricular is often disastrous, so, if in doubt, always assume you are dealing with a ventricular tachycardia. Electrophysiological studies, the ultimate arbiter of a tachycardia's origin, show that the majority of wide complex tachycardias are indeed ventricular in origin.

(2) DC reversion, the treatment of choice, is almost always effective. If it is not, check that the patient is not hypoxic, anxious or in pain or electrolytically unbalanced. If you do not have the equipment, or DC reversion is unsuccessful, use drugs as for ventricular ectopics. If the situation is deteriorating, con-

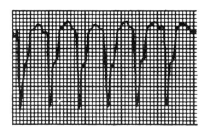

Fig. 11 There is no easily discernible P wave in this recording and it is impossible to tell whether this is supraventricular tachycardia with bundle branch block or ventricular tachycardia.

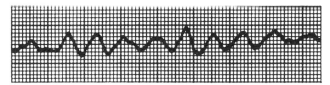

Fig. 12 Ventricular fibrillation.

tact a specialist unit for advice. They may be able to offer either paired or coupled pacing.

(3) If you have to use a drug in circumstances in which you are not sure of the origin of the arrhythmia, use amiodarone.

(4) Digoxin should never be used in patients with ventricular arrhythmias.

(5) Following the correction of a ventricular arrhythmia, give lignocaine i.v. for 24 h (see p. 18), in the expectation that this will prevent further episodes.

Ventricular fibrillation (see Fig. 12)
This is, of course, one of the causes of cardiac arrest. Its treatment is outlined on p. 3.

HEART BLOCK

This takes one of the following forms.

(1) First degree. This is defined as a P-R interval prolonged for more than 0.22 s (Fig. 13). This occurs in digoxin overdosage,

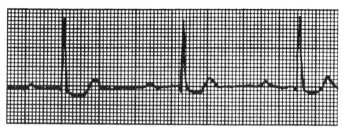

Fig. 13 First degree heart block. The P–R interval is greatly prolonged to 0.36 s.

coronary artery disease, myocarditis and excessive vagal tone. It is of little significance and is not treated unless:

(a)   it lengthens, and/or
(b)   dropped beats start to occur.

Either may herald complete heart block and if (a) and (b) occurs following a myocardial infarct, insertion of a temporary transvenous pacemaker should be considered.[3]

(2) Second degree. Here the ventricles do not always respond to atrial contraction. There are two types of second degree block, first clearly distinguished by Mobitz, and designated Mobitz type I and type II.

   (i)   Mobitz type I. In this type of block there is a progressively lengthening P-R interval culminating in a dropped beat (the Wenckebach phenomenon, Fig. 14) or the conducted beat has a prolonged P-R interval (Fig. 15a). The prognosis of Mobitz type I block is good and normal conduction may often be restored with atropine 0.6–2.4 mg i.v. or, failing this, dopamine (see p. 16). If these fail, or the patient's output is compromised or the degree of block progresses, a pacemaker should be inserted.

   (ii)   Mobitz type II. Here the conducted beat has a normal P-R interval (Fig. 15b). The ratio between non-conducted atrial contractions may be as great as 5 : 1. Since Mobitz type II block often progresses to complete heart block, a transvenous pacemaker should be inserted

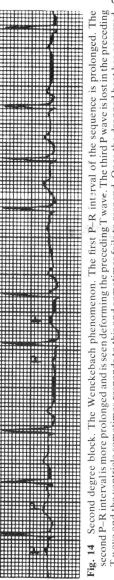

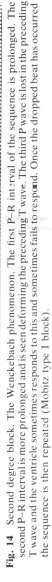

Fig. 14 Second degree block. The Wenckebach phenomenon. The first P–R interval of the sequence is prolonged. The second P–R interval is more prolonged and is seen deforming the preceding T wave. The third P wave is lost in the preceding T wave and the ventricle sometimes responds to this and sometimes fails to respond. Once the dropped beat has occurred the sequence is then repeated (Mobitz type I block).

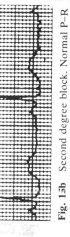

Fig. 15b Second degree block. Normal P–R interval of conducted beat (Mobitz type II block).

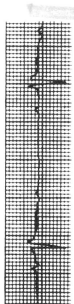

Fig. 15a Second degree block. Prolonged P–R interval of conducted beat (Mobitz type I block).

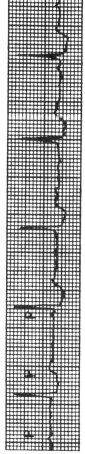

Fig. 16 Complete heart block. The first three P waves are marked. They can be seen to be beating quite independently of the QRS complex.

as soon as possible. Sympathomimetic agents should be used with care in this type of block, as an increase in atrial rate may increase the ratio of atrial to ventricular beats, causing the ventricular rate to slow. Use atropine whilst getting ready to pace your patient.

(3) Complete heart block (Fig. 16). Here the ventricular activity bears no temporal relationship to atrial activity. It is usually due to fibrous replacement of the conducting system, but may occur after myocardial infarction. It may rarely be caused by digoxin toxicity, or trauma to the bundle of His (e.g. after cardiac surgery).

Complete heart block may:

(i)   cause congestive cardiac failure,
(ii)   cause hypotension and poor tissue perfusion,
(iii) be punctuated by attacks of ventricular asystole, tachycardia or VF (Stokes–Adams attacks).

Treatment of complete heart block

(1) When this occurs following myocardial infarction, a temporary transvenous pacemaker should be inserted immediately, under fluoroscopic control.[3] Sinus rhythm usually returns within 1 week of infarction, but may take up to 3. If it does not, permanent pacing will be required.

(2) In other circumstances, if the low heart rate is causing symptoms, a permanent pacemaker should be inserted, if necessary preceded by a temporary wire as in (1) above. If pacing is not available, or while things are being organised, either give i.v. dopamine (see p. 16) or alternatively 2 mg isoprenaline in 500 ml of dextrose infused at a rate of 3–8 μg (10–30 drops)/min, until the ventricular rate is above 60 beats/min.

(3) Complete heart block may be presaged by the following.[10]

(i)   A lesser degree of block (see p. 33).
(ii)   A combination of left axis deviation (signifying left anterior hemiblock) and right bundle branch block (RBBB, Fig. 17), or right axis deviation (signifying left posterior hemiblock) and right bundle branch block (Fig. 18). Both of these configurations imply that at least two out of three of the conducting bundles are damaged, some of these patients progressing to complete block, as may patients developing left bundle branch block (LBBB) following myocardial infarction.[4,8]

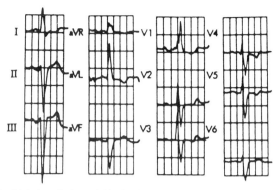

Fig. 17 Right bundle branch block with left axis deviation. (Reproduced, with permission, from Stock J. P. P. and Williams D. O. (1974). *Diagnosis and Treatment of Cardiac Arrhythmias.* London: Butterworths.)

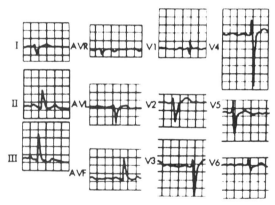

Fig. 18 Right bundle branch block with right axis deviation. (Reproduced, with permission, from Stock J. P. P. and Williams D. O. (1974). *Diagnosis and Treatment of Cardiac Arrhythmias.* London: Butterworths.)

(iii) The ECG configurations in (i) and (ii) above, or the development of LBBB, are an indication for pacing if:

    (a) they develop after an anterior wall myocardial infarction;

    (b) they are associated with symptoms attributable to Stokes–Adams attacks.

REFERENCES

General

Aronson J. K. (1985). Cardiac arrhythmias; theory and practice. *Br. Med. J.*; **290:** 487.

Hart G. *et al.* (1985). Physiology of cardiac conduction. *Br. J. Hosp. Med.*; **32:** 128.

Hillis W., Whiting B. (1983). Antiarrhythmic drugs. *Br. Med. J.*; **286:** 1332.

Schamroth L. (1971). *The Disorders of Cardiac Rhythm.* Oxford: Blackwell Scientific.

Specific

1 Blandford R. L. (1982). Intravenous amiodarone in atrial fibrillation complicating myocardial infarction. *Br. Med. J.*; **284:** 16.

2 Campbell D. R. (1983). Treatment and prophylaxis of ventricular arrhythmias in acute myocardial infarction. *Am. J. Cardiol.*; **52:** 55.

3 Harris A. N. (1969). Transvenous pacing. *Br. J. Hosp. Med.*; **2:** 1131.

4 Hollander G. *et al.* (1983). Bundle branch block in acute myocardial infarction. *Am. Heart J.*; **105:** 738.

5 Koch-Weser J. (1979). Disopyramide. *N. Engl. J. Med.*; **300:** 957.

6 Leader (1977). Sick sinus syndrome. *Br. Med. J.*; **1:** 4.

7 Leader (1981). Clinical implications of the diving response. *Lancet*; **i:** 1403.

8 McAnulty J. *et al.* (1982). Natural history of 'high risk' bundle branch block. *N. Engl. J. Med.*; **307:** 137.

9 Schamroth L. *et al.* (1972). Immediate effect of i.v. verapamil in cardiac arrhythmias. *Br. Med. J.*; **1:** 660.

10 Sclarovsky S. *et. al.* (1984). Advanced early and late atrioventricular block in acute inferior wall myocardial infarction. *Am. Heart J.*; **108:** 19.

11 Selzer A. S. (1982). Atrial fibrillation revisited. *N. Engl. J. Med.*; **306:** 1044.

Acute pulmonary oedema

DIAGNOSIS

(1) Acute pulmonary oedema is usually caused by a rise in pulmonary capillary pressure overcoming the osmotic pressure of plasma proteins. The rise in pulmonary capillary pressure is usually caused by left ventricular failure, in which case the following factors pertain.

   (i)   There is usually a history of increasing dyspnoea, fatigue, anorexia and orthopnoea, which may be accompanied by a dry cough and possibly attacks of paroxysmal nocturnal dyspnoea with production of pink frothy sputum.

   (ii)   Examination reveals a frightened, gasping patient who is pale and cyanosed with cold peripheries and who is pouring with sweat. The arterial pressure may be high, with a narrow pulse pressure, and in addition pulsus alternans may be present. A third heart sound and loud P2 may be present but are usually difficult to hear because of lung sounds—there are widespread loud crackles and wheezes over the lung fields. The sputum is pink and frothy.

   (iii) The chest x-ray is characteristic, with semiconfluent mottling spreading from the hila, and enlarged upper lobe pulmonary veins. In addition there may be left ventricular enlargement, Kerley 'B' lines and pleural effusions. The left ventricular end-diastolic pressure will be raised (see (iv) and (v) below). There may also be evidence of an obvious cause.

   (iv) The pulmonary capillary pressure (PCP) at which pulmonary oedema secondary to left ventricular failure occurs depends on the serum albumin level. At a normal serum albumin level of 32 g/l, pulmonary oedema due to heart failure will only occur when the PCP is above 25 mmHg. At lower albumin concentrations, pulmonary oedema will occur when the PCP is less than 18 mmHg. A simple formula (serum albumin (g/l) $\times$ 0.57 expressed as mmHg) gives an approximation to this critical pressure (but see p. 298).

(v)   The PCP is essentially the same as the left atrial pressure (which in its turn reflects the left ventricular end-diastolic pressure). The left atrial pressure is usually measured indirectly using a Swan–Ganz catheter with its tip wedged in a small pulmonary artery (see p. 347).

(2) Pulmonary oedema can also occur in patients who are severely ill for other reasons (e.g. septicaemia, acute renal failure) and who do not have a raised left atrial pressure. Here the likely cause is transudation of fluid from damaged capillaries. The appearance and management of these patients differ from those of the patient in left ventricular failure (see section on shock lung, p. 91).

(3) Acute pulmonary oedema has to be distinguished from the following.

(i)   Asthma (see p. 75). In both conditions the patient prefers sitting up, tachycardia is present, and both may give rise to inverted T waves on the ECG. In asthma there is more high-pitched wheeze and fewer crackles than in acute pulmonary oedema. The patient is not grey and sweaty unless in extremis, when parts of the lung fields are virtually silent; there is a quick inspiratory snatch and a prolonged expiratory phase; pulsus paradoxus may be present; the sputum is white and very sticky; the chest x-ray is usually normal or shows hyperinflation of the lungs. When, as sometimes happens, the main clinical evidence for pulmonary oedema is wheezing, the clinical situation and chest x-ray help distinguish it from asthma.

(ii) Pulmonary embolus (see p. 47).

(iii) Acute or chronic respiratory failure may mimic acute pulmonary oedema and be preceded by a history of orthopnoea. Measurement of Pa_{CO_2} before morphine and oxygen are given may help distinguish between the two, and must be made if there is any doubt. Unfortunately, patients who have no pre-existing lung disease may sometimes have a raised Pa_{CO_2} when in LVF.[1]

(iv) Other causes of acute shortness of breath (see p. 335) which are less easily confused.

(4) The causes of pulmonary oedema must be considered, especially the following treatable conditions.

(i)   Myocardial infarction (see p. 10).
(ii)   Severe hypertension (see p. 44).
(ii)   Mitral stenosis and regurgitation, aortic stenosis and cardiac aneurysms.
(iv)   Subacute bacterial endocarditis.
(v)   Cardiac arrhythmias (see p. 23).
(vi)   Water and salt overload, especially in an anuric patient.
(vii)   Pulmonary embolus. This may so compromise oxygen supply to the heart that left ventricular failure develops.
(viii) Cardiac tamponade.
(ix)   Cardiomyopathy.
(x)   Left atrial myxoma or ball valve thrombus (once in a lifetime).

MANAGEMENT

Management involves reducing the pulmonary oedema as follows.

(1) Sit the patient up if he has not already done so himself, either in a cardiac bed or with the legs over the side of the bed.
(2) Give the following.

   (i)   *Oxygen*, by either MC mask or nasal catheter, 4–6 l/min. If the patient has chronic respiratory failure, give 24% O_2 initially by a Ventimask. If the PaO_2 is less than 40 mmHg (5.3 kPa), increase the percentage of oxygen whilst monitoring the PaCO_2 (see p. 71).
   (ii)   *Morphine* 5–10 mg and an *antiemetic* such as cyclizine 50 mg i.v. If the patient has chronic respiratory failure, there is no safe sedation. If he is very distressed, probably the best thing to do is to give a small dose of morphine together with doxapram (1 mg/kg i.v.) and treat respiratory depression as necessary, whilst monitoring the blood gases.
   (iii) *Frusemide* 40 mg i.v.
   (iv)   *Aminophylline*, which helps to reduce bronchospasm and in addition may lower the pulmonary venous pressure. A loading dose of 5 mg/kg slowly over 30 min followed by an infusion at 0.5 mg/kg per h attains adequate blood levels safely, but may occasionally cause headaches and nausea. The dose may need modifying in old or very ill patients (see p. 77).

    (v)   *A cardiac glycoside.* If the patient has not had a cardiac glycoside within the last 5 days, give ouabain, a rapid-acting cardiac glycoside with a half-life of about 21 h. The dose is 0.5–1.0 mg i.v. slowly, repeated 4-hourly as necessary to a maximum of 2.0 mg in 24 h. The patient may later be transferred to digoxin (0.125–0.5 mg daily depending on size, age and renal function) for mainte-nance.

    (vi)   *Glyceryl trinitrate.* This venodilator reduces preload, and hence left ventricular end-diastolic pressure; 0.5 mg sub-lingually is an important adjunct to therapy.

(3) Having given (ii)–(vi) above, reassure the patient and then leave the nurse to make observations. Do not hover looking anxious; this will increase the patient's anxiety.

(4) If, three-quarters of an hour later, the patient is:

    (i)   the same:

        (a) repeat the dose of frusemide,
        (b) give a further 5 mg of morphine, both i.v.;

    (ii)   worse:

        (a) let 1 pint (0.6 litres) of blood—this is best done with an ordinary blood donor's set;
        (b) cuffing the limbs is now known to be ineffective in LVF.[2]

(5) If, despite these measures, the patient continues to deteriorate, consider putting him on a ventilator. Positive pressure venti-lation will reduce the venous return, lower the arterial pressure, and force the oedema back out of the alveoli. This may hold the situation until the other measures have taken effect.

INVESTIGATION AND TREATMENT OF THE CAUSE

(1) A chest x-ray and ECG should be taken as soon as possible.

(2) If an arrhythmia is thought to be the cause, the ECG should be continuously displayed on an oscilloscope. The arrhythmia is treated in the usual way (see p. 23). In particular, atrial fibril-lation may be an important contributory cause in an already jeopardised myocardium.

(3) Many patients with acute pulmonary oedema have a transiently elevated arterial pressure. However, if there is evidence of previous hypertension (hypertensive retinopathy, left ventricular hypertrophy and the diastolic pressure is maintained at >110 mmHg), steps should be taken to lower it (see p. 45).

(4) Acute pulmonary oedema in the following settings may require treatment as indicated.

(i) Mitral stenosis is an indication for an emergency valvotomy if the patient is already on adequate medical treatment.

(ii) Anuria is an absolute indication for dialysis.

(iii) Papillary muscle and ventricular septa can rupture following myocardial infarction and may be amenable to surgical repair.

(iv) Cardiac tamponade is an indication for paracentesis of the effusion without delay.

(v) A cardiac aneurysm: intractable cardiac failure may be controlled by resection of the redundant muscle.

(vi) Atrial myxoma or ball valve thrombus can be relieved, it is said, by repositioning the patient, head down.

REFERENCES

1   Leader (1972). Blood gas tensions in acute pulmonary oedema. *Lancet*; **i:** 1106.
2   Leader (1975). Rotating tourniquets for left ventricular failure. *Lancet*; **i:** 154.

Hypertension

(1) Hypertension may be regarded as an emergency in the following situations.

    (i)   When it is causing left ventricular failure (see p. 39).

    (ii)   When it is causing hypertensive encephalopathy.[5] This causes periodic attacks of severe headache, accompanied by vomiting, convulsions, confusion, deterioration of vision, possibly focal neurological signs and eventually coma. On examination the systolic and diastolic arterial pressures are usually more than 200 mmHg and 140 mmHg respectively. The fundus shows florid hypertensive changes and the urine contains protein. Treatment is by reduction of the arterial pressure (see p. 45).

    (iii) When it occurs in association with dissections of an aortic aneurysm (see p. 58).

    (iv) In accelerated or malignant hypertension. Here there are retinal haemorrhages and proteinuria, and the diastolic arterial pressure is usually above 120 mmHg.

    (v)   When it occurs in association with acute or chronic renal failure (see p. 139).

    (vi) In eclampsia and pre-eclampsia.

(2) There are three common pitfalls where a high arterial pressure reading is given in a situation which does not in itself require treatment.

    (i)   A single arterial pressure reading taken shortly after first meeting a patient. The patient's outward calm may be belied by the accompanying tachycardia.

    (ii)   When the arterial pressure reading is artificially elevated by gross obesity.

    (iii) When the systolic pressure is elevated by a rigid atheromatous aorta.

(3) The effect of a high arterial pressure can be seen directly in the fundus and can be inferred from the following clinical and ECG evidence.

    (i)   Deepest S wave in right ventricular leads plus tallest R wave in left ventricular leads add up to more than 36 mm.

(ii)   ST depression plus T wave inversion in left ventricular leads.

(4)   There are dangers in lowering blood pressure acutely, particularly in the elderly where too rapid reduction may compromise cerebral renal or myocardial blood flow. Only in categories (ii), (iii), (v) and (vi) above do we recommend i.v. therapy. In other circumstances, oral therapy can be used.

MANAGEMENT

Reduction of diastolic arterial pressure to 100 mmHg is all that should be attempted. Further reduction may reduce cerebral blood flow to such an extent that neurological symptoms occur. Special care is needed in treating patients who have cerebral infarction with associated severe hypertension (see p. 193).

The arterial pressure may be lowered rapidly with any one of the following.

(1)   Sodium nitroprusside.[6] This is the drug of choice. If your pharmacy has no access to the ready-made solutions, make up a fresh solution of 50 mg sodium nitroprusside in 500 ml of 5% dextrose (0.01% solutions). This is given continuously i.v. An incremental infusion rate in the dose range 0.5–10.0 μg/kg per min may be required for short periods of time. It is mandatory to measure thiocyanate and cyanide levels with exceptionally high doses, but at doses of under 10 μg/kg per min no adverse side-effects have been noted.[6] Cyanide poisoning can be reversed by giving hydroxycyanocobalamin 1000 μg i.v. or, in severe cases, the specific antidote to cyanide poisoning, dicobalt EDTA in a dose of 300 mg i.v.

(2)   Hydralazine.[4] Give 10 mg i.v. or i.m. The dose may be repeated every 30 min as necessary. Common toxic effects are tachycardia, headaches, nausea and vomiting. Occasional dizziness, flushing and sweating, dyspnoea, angina, paraesthesiae and urticaria may occur.

(3)   Diazoxide.[3] Give 5 mg/kg rapidly i.v. The dose may be repeated as necessary. Side-effects are the development of hyperglycaemia and sodium and water retention.

Hydralazine and diazoxide both increase cardiac stroke volume and cardiac work; thus, in patients with dissecting aneurysm or with pulmonary oedema sodium nitroprusside is preferable.

(4) Oral therapy. A combination of a β-blocker (such as atenolol 100 mg) and a diuretic (bendrofluazide 5–10 mg) produces a smooth fall in arterial pressure over 12–24 h, and is often all that is required. An alternative is nifedipine 10 mg orally, which starts to lower blood pressure within 10 min and has a maximal action within 30–40 min. The dose can then be repeated as required to keep the blood pressure down. We use this with increasing frequency as it seems to preserve cerebral blood flow well, so it combines safety with convenience, particularly where monitoring facilities are not readily available.[1]

(5) If you do use i.v. therapy, treatment with diuretics in doses adequate to maintain urinary output, and oral hypotensives should start at the same time.

(6) Hypertensive crisis in phaeochromocytoma must be treated with an α-adrenergic blocking drug. Give phentolamine 2.5–5.0 mg i.v. at 5 min intervals until the arterial pressure is controlled and thereafter at 2–4 h intervals, or as needed to keep the arterial pressure under control.

Phentolamine may also be given as a continuous infusion at a rate of 0.2–0.5 mg/mm. Sodium nitroprusside may also be used in this situation.

(7) Hypertensive crisis in pregnancy. In the UK hydralazine is the drug with which we have the most experience, given as outlined in (2) above.

REFERENCES

1 Bertel O. *et al.* (1983). Nifedipine in hypertensive emergencies. *Br. Med. J.*; **286:** 19.

2 Koch-Weser J. (1974). Hypertensive emergencies. *N. Engl. J. Med.*; **290:** 211.

3 Koch-Weser J. (1976). Diazoxide. *N. Engl. J. Med.*; **294:** 1271.

4 Koch-Weser J. (1976). Hydralazine. *N. Engl. J. Med.*; **295:** 320.

5 Leader (1979). Hypertensive encephalopathy. *Br. Med. J.*; **2:** 1387.

6 Palmer R. F., Lasseter K. C. (1975). Sodium nitroprusside. *N. Engl. J. Med.*; **292:** 294.

Pulmonary embolus [1,7,8,9]

DIAGNOSIS

(1) Pulmonary embolus, depending on its size, may present as one of four clinical pictures, the last three of which may overlap to some extent.

Group A. Sudden death. The diagnosis is established at post mortem.

Group B. Acute dyspnoea, which occurs in 70% of patients in this group, is accompanied by syncope or collapse in 80%, and central chest pain in 35%. This needs to be distinguished from myocardial infarction (see below).

Group C. Pleuritic pain and haemoptysis, unaccompanied by signs of circulatory failure. This needs to be distinguished from pneumonia (see below).

Group D. Shortness of breath alone. This characteristically insidious onset of multiple pulmonary emboli should always be considered in a patient with a history of slowly progressive dyspnoea.

(2) The signs on examination will again vary according to the size of the embolus.

(i) The signs of pulmonary hypertension may be present if approximately two-thirds of the area of the pulmonary arterial bed is obstructed. These signs, which occur in a major pulmonary embolus (group B above), include:

(a) a giant 'a' wave in the jugular venous pulse,
(b) a powerful parasternal heave,
(c) a right atrial gallop (triple heart sounds heard loudest in the pulmonary area),
(d) accentuation of the pulmonary second sound,
(e) tachypnoea, tachycardia, cyanosis and hypotension are also frequently present.

(ii) The signs of pulmonary infarction. This does not invariably follow pulmonary embolus but is usually present if pleuritic pain occurs—characteristically group C. A

47

pleural friction rub is heard and if the infarct is large, this is followed in about 48 h by dullness, decreased breath sounds and crackles over the site of the infarct.

(3) The legs should always be examined for signs of deep vein thrombosis (DVT).[11-13] These thrombi, of course, are the source of the embolus.

The signs are:

(i)   delayed cooling of the exposed leg, and
(ii) increased size of the calf, the careful measurement of which should be compared with the other leg.

These are two of the most reliable signs of deep vein thrombosis. In addition there may be:

(i)   accentuation of the venous pattern and oedema of the ankle and foot,
(ii)   tenderness on palpation of the calf muscles or Hunter's canal,
(iii) the presence of thrombi in the veins above the knee (the usual source of emboli) which can be confirmed simply by ultrasound and impedance plethysmography.

The absence of DVT does not exclude a pulmonary embolus—all the clot may have travelled to the lung by the time of your investigations.

Remember that Homan's sign is falsely positive or falsely negative too often to be of any value, and that 70% of DVTs give rise to neither signs nor symptoms.

(4) Investigations include the following.

(i)   Chest x-ray. Frequently there may be no evidence of large pulmonary emboli on an ordinary chest x-ray. Collapse of part of a lung may be inferred from an elevated diaphragm (the first sign to develop) and increased translucency of one lobe or lung. As the infarct becomes haemorrhagic the characteristic wedge-shaped shadow appears. In addition, the pulmonary artery diameter may be enlarged (more than 17 mm in a man and more than 16 mm in a woman) or the pulmonary artery may even be seen to terminate abruptly—'pulmonary cut off'.
(ii)   ECG. The ECG may be initially normal, but may change rapidly in the early phases of the illness. Characteristic patterns of change are as follows.

I II III   aVR aVL aVF

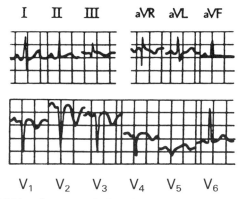

V₁ V₂ V₃ V₄ V₅ V₆

Fig. 19 ECG in pulmonary embolism. (Reproduced, with permission, from Oram S. (1984). *Clinical Heart Disease* 2nd edn. London: Heinemann Medical.)

(a) An attempt to develop right axis deviation (an S wave in I), a Q wave in III with a raised ST segment and inverted T wave (but not also in II as in inferior myocardial infarction) and inverted T waves across the right ventricular chest leads with clockwise rotation (Fig. 19).

(b) Development of right bundle branch block.

(c) Any of the conventional ischaemic patterns, presumably provoked by low coronary artery blood flow.

(iii) A perfusion scan of the lungs may reveal areas of diminished flow at a time when chest x-ray is normal. In a person with pre-existing lung disease, it is helpful to combine the perfusion scan with a ventilation scan. A gross mismatch, showing underperfusion of normally ventilated areas is characteristic of pulmonary embolism.[15]

(iv) Arterial blood gases. The Pa_{O_2} is usually below 60 mmHg (8.0 kPa) in substantial embolisation.

(v) Pulmonary arteriography is the only certain way of diagnosing pulmonary embolus. It may demonstrate absent or incomplete filling of the pulmonary vasculature. The indications for this investigation (which is quick and is of minimal inconvenience to the patient if the specialised equipment and experience are available) are discussed below. Retrograde venography undertaken at the same time may show the source of the embolus in the pelvic or leg veins.[2] Digital vascular imaging (DVI), using low doses of contrast medium through central lines, is an exciting new diagnostic technique.

(vi) Bilirubin, lactic dehydrogenase (LDH) and transaminase levels are seldom diagnostically helpful.

MANAGEMENT

Group A is fatal by definition. Group B is frequently fatal. Group C should always be treated urgently because some 30% of patients who survive one embolus have a second, which is fatal in about 20% of cases. Patients in group D also require urgent treatment but are not, unlike groups B and C, in mortal danger.

Management involves the following.

(1) Establishing the diagnosis. As indicated above, physical examination of the acute case may be helpful, but is seldom conclusive. Additional information is needed from the chest x-ray and ECG, which should both be obtained as soon as possible. Pulmonary arteriography, being the only certain diagnostic measure, should be undertaken in any patient in whom there is clinical suspicion of a major pulmonary embolus. The radio-opaque dye used during arteriography is a vaso-dilator. Give phenylephrine 0.1–0.5 mg i.v. immediately prior to the examination in order to forestall a catastrophic fall in arterial pressure. (The lower dose of dye used in DVI makes this unnecessary when this mode of investigation is used.)

(2) Restoring the systemic circulation. This is the first considera-tion in group B and is most effectively achieved by moving the embolus. How to do this is controversial, but the following factors are relevant.

(i) If the heart has stopped, cardiac massage may not only restart it but may also break up and disperse the embolus.

(ii) If the patient is in shock or deteriorating rapidly with signs of progressive right heart failure, and is not respond-ing to, or not able to have fibrinolytics, pulmonary embo.ectomy should be undertaken. Heparin should then be used postoperatively. In less grave situations a trial of fibrinolytic therapy is justified.

(iii) Thrombolytics (fibrinolytics) may be infused into the pulmonary arteries through the catheter with which the arteriogram has been done.[14] These agents are plasminogen activators; the plasmin so generated is a proteolytic enzyme. By digesting fibrin, it dissolves clots. If your patient has active gastrointestinal bleeding, or has had a stroke within the past 2 months, these agents are absolutely contraindicated. Relative contraindications include major surgery, obstetrical delivery, organ biopsy, gastrointestinal (GI) bleed or serious trauma within the previous 10 days. A systolic arterial pressure of >200 mmHg, or diastolic arterial pressure of >110 mmHg is another relative contraindication.

Give either urokinase or streptokinase.

(a) Urokinase (which is expensive but not allergenic) 4400 i.u./kg over 10 min, and then 4400 i.u./kg per hour for 24 h. If the initial response is unsatisfactory, continue the infusion at the same rate to a total of 700 000 units.

(b) Streptokinase (which is cheaper, but is allergenic). Give an initial dose of 250 000 units in 30 min and then infuse 100 000 units/h for 24 h.

Both these are hazardous, in that severe bleeding may occur during the infusion. To minimise the chances of bleeding, you should:

minimise the physical handling of the patient,
discontinue parenteral medicine wherever possible, and substitute appropriate oral therapy,
minimise all invasive procedures,
apply compression bandages at the site of vessel punctures,
avoid concurrent anticoagulation, or treatment with antiplatelet drugs.

If bleeding does occur, stop the fibrinolytic agent (the half-life of which is usually only 0.5 h), and give fresh whole blood. Failing this, give fresh frozen plasma and cryoprecipitate to replace the fibrinogen and other coagulation factors. Epsilon aminocaproic acid, in a dose of 5 g, can be given in the rare event of the above measures being unsuccessful.

(iv) Monitoring fibrinolytic therapy. The best way to do this is by measuring the whole blood euglobin lysis time, the next best is the thrombin time. These are not generally available, and the partial thromboplastin time is a reasonable alternative. Take a preinfusion control value, and repeat 4 h after the infusion has started. If the PTT is increased, you can assume that systemic lysis has been achieved.

(v) After completing the thrombolytic therapy, a continuous infusion of heparin should be started as soon as the PTT falls to less than twice the control value.[12]

(vi) While definitive measures are being initiated, you may have to support the circulation. To this end, it is important to keep the right atrial pressure (and thus the right ventricular filling pressure) high. A pressure of 12 mmHg above the sternal angle appears to be optimal for maximising right-sided stroke work in this situation. The right atrial pressure tends to be high anyway in major pulmonary emboli but if less than 12 mmHg, infuse Haemaccel or dextran 70 under CVP control. You will probably only need a few hundred millilitres so be wary.

If raising the right ventricular filling pressure is to no avail, use inotropic agents (see p. 16).

(3) Reversing hypoxia, which is always present because intrapulmonary shunting, alveolar hypoventilation, and impaired perfusion occur.[3] Oxygen via an MC mask is partly effective in relieving this hypoxia.

(4) Relieving pain. Give diamorphine (see p. 11).

(5) In groups C and D the systemic circulation is not jeopardised and none of the measures (i)–(iii) is required. However, in all groups, whatever the initial treatment, further emboli can be prevented by anticoagulants, and this treatment should be undertaken as indicated on p. 17.

(6) Removal or exclusion of any remaining deep vein thrombi These have first to be identified, either by retrograde phlebography at the same time as the pulmonary arteriogram, or by bilateral ascending femoral phlebography. After identification either direct surgical removal or proximal ligation of the affected vein can be undertaken, depending on the site of the thrombus. An alternative is to infuse fibrinolytic agents locally or systemically, in the doses given above.[6]

Pregnancy

In the particular circumstances of pulmonary embolism in pregnancy, anticoagulation should be commenced with heparin, as advocated on p. 17. Warfarin is best not used since it is teratogenic and is also associated with an increased incidence of antepartum haemorrhage.[5]

Remember that the prevention of venous thrombosis is the key to the prevention of pulmonary embolism.[4,10]

REFERENCES

1   Adelstein J. S. (1978). A new diagnostic tool for pulmonary embolus. How good and how costly? *N. Engl. J. Med.*; **299:** 305.

2   Dow J. D. (1973). Retrograde phlebography in major PE. *Lancet*; **ii:** 407.

3   Hayes S. P., Bone R. C. (1983). Pulmonary emboli with respiratory failure. *Med. Clin. N. Am.*; **67:** 1179.

4   Leader (1975). Low dose heparin and the prevention of thrombo-embolic disease. *Br. Med. J.*; **3:** 447.

5   Leader (1979). Thrombo-embolism in pregnancy. *Br. Med. J.*; **1:** 1661.

6   Leader (1981). Streptokinase and deep venous thrombosis. *Lancet*; **i:** 1035.

7   Miller J. A. H. (1972). Diagnosis and management of massive pulmonary embolus. *Br. J. Surg.*; **59:** 837.

8   Oakley C. M. (1970). Diagnosis of pulmonary embolism. *Br. Med. J.*; **2:** 773.

9   Ruckley C. V. (1982). Management of pulmonary embolism. *Br. Med. J.*; **285:** 831.

10 Salzman E. W. (1983). Progress in preventing venous thrombo-embolism. *N. Engl. J. Med.*; **309:** 980.

11 Salzman E. W. (1986). Venous thrombosis made easy. *N. Engl. J. Med.*; **314:** 847.

12 Salzman E. W. *et al.* (1975). Management of heparin therapy. *N. Engl. J. Med.*; **292:** 1045.

13 Sandler D. A. *et al.* (1984). Diagnosis of deep venous thrombosis: comparison of clinical evaluation, ultrasound, plethysmograph, and venoscan with X-ray venogram. *Lancet*; **ii:** 716.

14 Sharma G. V. R. K. (1982). Thrombolytic therapy: *N. Engl. J. Med.*; **306:** 1268.

15   Spies W. B. *et al.* (1986). Ventilation/perfusion scintigraphy in suspected pulmonary embolus, correlation with pulmonary angiography and refinement of criteria of interpretation. *Radiology*; **159:** 383.

Peripheral embolus [1,2,3,4]

DIAGNOSIS

Obstruction of blood supply to an organ usually causes a sudden onset of severe pain, numbness and loss of function. The basis for obstruction is usually either embolus or local thrombosis. It may be impossible to decide between the two but, fortunately, therapy is similar.

The diagnosis should be considered in anyone in whom the above-mentioned symptoms occur, especially when there is an obvious source of embolus, e.g. recent myocardial infarction, atrial fibrillation, mitral stenosis. Thus, the following diagnostic factors should be sought.

(1) In the limbs. The patient complains of coldness and/or pain. On examination the limb is pale and cold and the peripheral pulses are absent. The diagnosis is usually fairly clear. However, it may be mimicked by a deep vein thrombosis which occurs in a leg with pre-existing obstructive arterial disease. Here also the leg is painful, pale and pulseless, but DVT may be differentiated from infarction by the development of oedema, which occurs only late in infarction. In addition an arterial embolus is experienced first as pain which passes into numbness.

(2) In the gut. Embolus causes abdominal pain with vomiting and possibly the passage of blood per rectum. There may be signs of peritonitis and impending intestinal obstruction. The patient rapidly deteriorates if infarction of bowel has occurred. Diagnosis is made at laparotomy.

(3) In the kidney. The patient complains of acute loin pain and haematuria, symptoms which may also be caused by a stone. An IVP and renogram should distinguish between these two, and an arterial occlusion can be confirmed by selective renal arteriography.

(4) In the carotid circulation. Embolus causes the onset of neurological signs, e.g. hemiplegia. If this occurs in a setting where an embolus is likely, early arteriography, preferably a DVI, should be undertaken to determine the site of the block.

Emboli are not infrequently multiple. All the peripheral pulses should be carefully palpated.

MANAGEMENT

(1) Control of pain with i.v. morphine (see p. 11).
(2) Conservation of the ischaemic area. This is only really possible in the limbs, which, pending definitive therapy, should be:

    (i)   exposed in a dependent position, and
    (ii)   cooled, using a portable fan.

(3) Minimising further thrombus formation. This is only practical in acute limb ischaemia, where you should give i.v. heparin (see p. 17), irrespective of whether you deem surgery likely or not. Anticoagulants may also prevent further emboli (see 5 below).
(4) Removal of the obstruction. As a general principle, this should be undertaken whenever possible.

    (i)   In the limbs. Surgery should be undertaken without delay, preferably after arteriography. The embolus may be removed under local anaesthetic. Therefore, the general condition of the patient is irrelevant, and a 'wait and see' policy is unjustified.

        If embolectomy is either unsuccessful or impossible, the following regimens may be helpful.

       (a) Alternate bottles of 20 ml 95% alcohol in 500 ml of saline with 500 ml dextran 70 in 5% dextrose 6-hourly.
       (b) Thrombolytic therapy (in doses as for pulmonary embolism) has been attended by successful dissolution of clot (see p. 51).
       (c) Adrenergic blocking agents are valueless.

    (ii)   In the gut. If at all possible, embolectomy and revascularisation of the bowel should be undertaken immediately. If infarction has occurred, survival without operation is extremely rare.
    (iii) In the kidney. Operation should be considered, at which either the embolus or the kidney is removed depending on the viability of the latter.
    (iv) In the extracranial carotid arteries. Immediate embolectomy under local anaesthetic may be considered.
    (v)   In the intracranial carotid arteries. Anticoagulants should be started after you have shown on CT scan that the infarct is not haemorrhagic.

(5) Prevention of further emboli. If the primary thrombus cannot be reached, a course of anticoagulants should be started (see p. 18) as they have been shown to reduce the incidence of further thrombi.

(6) Atrial fibrillation, which is often present, should be controlled with digitalis as necessary.

REFERENCES

1 Perrson A. V., Thomson J., Patman R. (1973). Streptokinase as an adjunct to arterial surgery. *Arch. Surg.*; **107:** 779.

2 Sewell I. A. (1985). Sudden arterial occlusion. *Hosp. Update*; **June:** 363.

3 Sewell I. A. (1985). Management of sudden arterial occlusion. *Hosp. Update*; **June:** 449.

4 Thompson J. E. (1980). Peripheral arterial surgery. *N. Engl. J. Med.*; **302:** 491.

Dissections of the aorta[1,2]

DIAGNOSIS

(1) The process of dissection may be intensely painful. Pain may be experienced in the chest, the back, the abdomen or the legs, depending upon the origin of the aneurysm; it may spread from one site to another, depending on the direction and extent of the dissection. In almost half the cases, however, pain is slight and the diagnosis is made from a chance finding on chest x-ray, from a sudden drop in the arterial pressure, or from the signs of ischaemia (see p. 55).

(2) The signs include the following.

(i) Shock (see p. 295), which may be due to severe pain or to loss of blood.

(ii) Signs of ischaemia in the:

(a) myocardium—myocardial infarction;
(b) limbs—apart from gross signs (see p. 55), a difference of 20 mmHg between the systolic arterial pressures of opposite limbs indicates arterial obstruction in the limb with the lower pressure;
(c) brain—a hemi- or quadriplegia;
(d) kidneys—if both kidneys are involved, as is usually the case, there is severe oliguria with a few red cells or complete anuria;
(e) gut (see p. 55);
(f) spinal cord—paraplegia.

(iii) Aortic regurgitation.
(iv) Haemopericardium.

(3) Investigations include the following.

(i) Chest x-ray. This should be repeated every 24 h in order to detect changes in the contour of the aorta.

(ii) Echocardiography. This may show widening of the aorta and the characteristic double lumen of the aorta. It cannot be used to exclude dissection but may provide useful positive information.

(iii) Aortography. This is the definitive investigation for a dissecting aortic aneurysm and must be undertaken if operative treatment is considered.

MANAGEMENT

The order of priorities of medical management is as follows.

(1) Relief of pain. Any one of the following combinations may be given and repeated as often as necessary provided the patient is not dangerously hypotensive.

    (i) Diamorphine 5–10 mg i.v. plus prochlorperazine 12.5 mg i.v.

    (ii) Morphine 15 mg i.v. plus prochlorperazine 12.5 mg i.v.

(2) Lowering the blood pressure if raised (see p. 45).
(3) Relief of cardiac tamponade (see p. 61).

Further management should be discussed with a cardiovascular surgeon who should be consulted as soon as the diagnosis has been considered.

REFERENCES

1   Godwin J. D. (1983). Acute diseases of the aorta. *Radiol. Clin. N. Am.*; **21:** 551.
2   Vecht R. J. *et al*. (1980). Acute dissection of the aorta: long term review and management: *Lancet*; **i:** 109.

Cardiac tamponade[1,3]

This term implies restriction of cardiac function by mechanical constriction of the heart. It is usually caused by a tense pericardial effusion or by a haemopericardium (which may follow a dissecting aneurysm, a chest injury or a myocardial infarction). It may also be caused by blood clots surrounding the heart, even when the pericardium has been left wide open, as after thoracic surgery.

DIAGNOSIS

(1) There may be a preceding history of precordial pain followed by increasing dyspnoea.

(2) The signs are as follows.

    (i) Decreased cardiac output. Despite a tachycardia, the patient is hypotensive, the pulse pressure is small and the peripheries are poorly perfused. In addition, pulsus paradoxus is usually present. This may be demonstrated by measuring the systolic arterial pressure in expiration and inspiration. If there is a fall of >10 mmHg on inspiration, then constriction is present.

    (ii) Increased pressure in the systemic and pulmonary veins. The jugular venous pressure is raised. The 'y' descent is rapid and there is a conspicuous 'y' trough. In addition, the jugular venous pressure rises on inspiration.

       Similarly, the respiratory rate is raised and the patient is occasionally orthopnoeic, with wheezes and possibly crackles in the chest.

    (iii) The effusion itself. It may be possible to demonstrate an increased area of dullness around the precordium. In addition, the apex beat is impalpable and the heart sounds are muffled. However, a third heart sound can usually be heard. Thus, the diagnosis should always be considered in a patient with severe left ventricular failure and/or hypotension.

    (iv) The above signs develop sequentially, over a variable time course. The progression seen serves as a useful guide to grading the severity of the effusion, as outlined below.

(a) *Grade 1.* JVP and heart rate are both increased, but cardiac output is normal.

(b) *Grade 2.* As above, with the addition of pulsus paradoxus and mild hypotension.

(c) *Grade 3.* As above, with in addition a poor cardiac output and muffling of the heart sounds.

(3) On screening, the cardiac outline is relatively immobile. The extent of the effusion may be estimated by cardiac catheterisation and angiography, echocardiography, or by a 'heart' scan with a radioisotope (technetium) tagged to the patient's red cells. The echocardiogram is the most reliable technique, and has the great advantage of being non-invasive.

(4) The ECG may be of low voltage and there may be widespread inversion of T waves.

(5) If cardiac tamponade needs to be relieved urgently, the signs are usually gross (i.e. Grade 3), the pulse almost disappearing on inspiration. The degree of severity may be caused by a surprisingly small effusion.

(6) Tamponade needs to be differentiated from other causes of a poor cardiac output with a raised JVP, importantly:

(i)   severe congestive cardiac failure.
(ii) pulmonary embolus (see p. 47).
(iii) right ventricular myocardial infarction (see p. 10).
(iv) superior venacaval obstruction: the immobility of the neck veins and suffusion of the face should help you here.

The distinction between these various categories is sometimes very difficult on clinical grounds. If you do not have echocardiogram facilities to help you, assume a pericardial effusion is present, and treat accordingly.

MANAGEMENT

(1) The heart must be decompressed:

(i)   if the patient is distressed,
(ii) if the systolic arterial pressure is <90 mmHg and/or the jugular venous pressure is more than 10 cmH$_2$O.

(2) If trauma is the cause of the tamponade, treatment is urgent thoracotomy. Pericardiocentesis, as outlined below, is, in this

circumstance, at best a holding manoeuvre, and should not delay surgery.

(3) In non-traumatic tamponade management is as follows.

(i) If the patient is in extremis, insert a wide-bore needle in the fourth intercostal space over the precordium and advance until fluid is obtained. This may release enough fluid—often surprisingly little—to relieve the heart.

(ii) Otherwise the site of choice is the xiphisternal angle. Sit the patient up at 45°, insert the needle 3 cm below the xiphisternum at an angle of between 30° and 45° to the skin. Apply suction to the needle, and push it slowly upwards and backwards until fluid is obtained, and then aspirate as much fluid as you can. The heart may be difficult to feel, but usually produces ectopic beats when scratched. If you have your needle connected to an ECG machine, as you should, you will get an appropriate recording (Fig. 20).

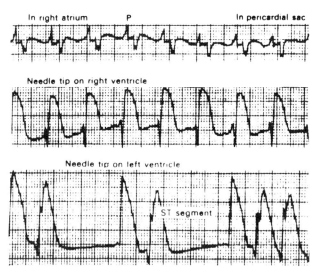

Fig. 20 Electrocardiogram obtained from the needle tip at three sites. (Reproduced with permission from Dr A. Hollman and the editors of *Medicine*.)

(iii) If the effusion is haemorrhagic, you may wonder if you have unwittingly entered a cardiac chamber. Place a few millilitres of the fluid in a glass tube: intracardiac blood will clot, haemorrhagic effusion will not.

(iv) To minimise the chances of your entering a cardiac chamber, it is helpful to attach your aspiration needle to the 'V' lead terminal on the ECG cable. This can be done by means of an insulated wire with a clip on each end; failing this, just attach the wire with Sellotape. Figure 20 shows the electrocardiograms obtained when the needle tip is advanced to three different sites.

(v) Both volume expansion and vasodilators have been advocated. There is good evidence that both are ineffective.[2]

REFERENCES

1   Callahan M. L. (1984). Pericardiocentesis in traumatic and non-traumatic cardiac tamponade. *Ann. Emer. Med.*; **13:** 924.

2   Kerber R. E. *et al.* (1982). Haemodynamic effects of volume expansion and nitroprusside compared with pericardiocentesis in patients with acute cardiac tamponade. *N. Engl. J. Med.*; **307:** 929.

3   Leader (1980). Cardiac tamponade. *Br. Med. J.*; **280:** 505.

SECTION II

RESPIRATORY

Respiratory failure[1]

DIAGNOSIS

(1) This is defined in terms of altered blood gases—an arterial oxygen tension (PaO$_2$) of less than 60 mmHg (8 kPa) with or without an arterial CO$_2$ tension (PaCO$_2$) of above 50 mmHg (6.7 kPa).

(2) Both hypoxia (low PaO$_2$) and hypercarbia (raised PaCO$_2$) are difficult to pick up clinically, for the following reasons.

    (i)   The classical signs of hypoxia are either non-specific (disturbances of consciousness, ranging from mild confusion to coma), or difficult to assess (cyanosis).

    (ii)   Hypercarbia may give rise to a spectrum of mental changes similar to those of hypoxia. It may also cause a flapping tremor, peripheral vasodilatation, papilloedema and early morning headaches, which again are not specific for a rising PaCO$_2$.

Hence arterial blood gas measurements are mandatory if the diagnosis is suspected.

There are three patterns for respiratory failure.

(1) *Pure ventilatory failure* which gives rise to a raised PaCO$_2$ and a low PaO$_2$. Examples of this are:

    (i)   depression of the respiratory centre by drugs,

    (ii)   neurological conditions such as poliomyelitis, myasthenia gravis, Guillain–Barré syndrome,

    (iii) primary alveolar hypoventilation (Pickwickian syndrome).

(2) *Hypoxaemic failure* due to local disturbances of the ventilation–perfusion relationship. This gives rise to a low PaO$_2$, with a low or normal PaO$_2$.[2] Examples of this are:

    (i)   'pure' emphysema,

    (ii)   asthma in the initial stages of an attack (see Fig. 21, p. 76),

    (iii) pneumonia (see p. 99),

(iv) left ventricular failure (but see p. 39),
(v)   fibrosing alveolitis,
(vi) shock lung (see p. 91).

(3) *A mixture of ventilatory and hypoxaemic failure.* This combination of alveolar hypoventilation and deranged ventilation–perfusion relationships produces a low Pa_{O_2}, with a raised Pa_{CO_2}. The example of this type of failure is chronic bronchitis with emphysema. Such patients frequently have a permanently low Pa_{O_2} and may have a permanently high Pa_{CO_2} (and therefore a high serum HCO_3). However, if, with a raised Pa_{CO_2}, the serum HCO_3 is relatively normal (below 30 mmol/l), and the pH is therefore low, the implications are that renal compensation has not occurred, and the respiratory failure has come on over a short time. This further implies that there are reversible elements, such as an acute infection with associated sputum retention, increasing airways obstruction and often heart failure. This is the commonest clinical setting for respiratory failure and the management of this is therefore discussed first.

ACUTE ON CHRONIC BRONCHITIS PRECIPITATING RESPIRATORY FAILURE

Diagnosis

(1) The patient often has a history of increasing breathlessness, increasing volumes of purulent sputum, and, occasionally, pleuritic pain. All this in the setting of chronic obstructive airways disease.
(2) Examination reveals a breathless, often pyrexial patient, who may be confused, cyanosed and have a tachycardia.
(3) There may be evidence of hypercarbia (see (2)(ii) above).
(4) There will be a prolonged expiratory phase, with variable crackles and wheezes.
(5) The signs of collapse, consolidation, effusion or pneumothorax must also be sought as any of these can exacerbate the situation.
(6) Signs of right-sided heart failure (raised neck veins, oedema and a palpable liver) are often present.

Management

Initial investigations, in order of priority, are as follows.

(1) Arterial blood gases and pH.
(2) Chest x-ray, most importantly to exclude a pneumothorax.
(3) Culture of sputum and blood.
(4) Knowledge of haemoglobin, electrolytes and urea, whereas not often immediately useful, will be required.

The aim of management is to increase intracellular O_2. Experience with tissue oxygen electrodes is limited and as yet this is usually measured indirectly by the $P\text{ao}_2$. The $P\text{ao}_2$ should be increased to at least 45 mmHg (6 kPa) and preferably to 50–55 mmHg (6.7–7.3 kPa), achieved preferably with a fall, or at least without a substantial rise, in the $P\text{aco}_2$.

Each of the factors (enumerated above) which contribute to the combination of ventilatory and hypoxaemic failure must be tackled.

(1) Infection. the commonest infecting organisms are *Streptococcus pneumoniae* and *Haemophilus influenzae*. Both are usually sensitive to amoxycillin 250 mg 8-hourly (parenterally or orally), tetracycline 500 mg 6-hourly (i.m. or orally, not i.v.) or cotrimoxazole tabs. ii b.d.

If the infection has been contracted in hospital, or if for other reasons you suspect that the infection may be caused by resistant staphylococci, add i.v. or i.m. flucloxacillin 500 mg 6-hourly.

If the sputum purulence has not decreased after 48 h, consider changing the antibiotic, but consult your bacteriologist first. Remember that sputum culture and sensitivity tests may be misleading, so do not change antibiotics exclusively on the basis of information from these.

(2) Sputum retention. A patient's outlook may be transformed if energetic and regular physiotherapy 'raises the sputum'. Initially physiotherapy must be given 2-hourly throughout the 24 h, and if necessary you must teach both day and night nurses how to give appropriate physiotherapy. The sputum should be loosened by clapping the chest for 3–4 min, after which the patient should take a few quick deep breaths and then cough. Ideally this should be done in appropriate bronchial drainage positions. This is rarely feasible, but at least place the patient first on one side and then on the other. If the patient is too confused to cooperate, give physiotherapy after nikethamide or doxapram. The sputum may be sticky, and intermittent humidification through a Wright's nebuliser can aid expectoration (4 ml of warm saline is as effective as anything and is

certainly cheapest). If despite these measures the patient still cannot bring up sputum, it must be sucked up by one of the following means.

(i) Nasotracheal suction. Sit the patient up and with a gloved hand pass a soft catheter with a round end (off suction lest the pharynx and trachea be traumatised) through a nostril and into the pharynx. A convenient arrangement for this is to attach the catheter to one limb of a Y connector, which is itself attached to a sucker. Suction is then applied by occluding the other limb. To be of maximum benefit, the catheter must pass between the cords. Encourage the patient to cough, and, as he exhales, advance the catheter and then suck

If the patient cannot phonate, you are probably through the cords. Advance the catheter into each main bronchus in turn. This is a potent stimulus to coughing and you should leave the catheter down until more sputum is forthcoming. If laryngospasm occurs, attempts to pass the catheter into the trachea should not be repeated.

(ii) Bronchoscopy. This should be undertaken if, despite nasotracheal suction, the patient continues to deteriorate, especially if the sputum retention produces lobar collapse. Flexible bronchoscopes have made this a much less traumatic event than previously and, given the circumstances, the patient's memory for the event is hazy.

(iii) Tracheal toilet through an endotracheal tube.

(3) Airways obstruction. The reversible component may be due to:

(i) sputum retention,
(ii) mucosal inflammation,
(iii) bronchospasm.

Treatments of (i) and (ii) have been discussed. Bronchospasm must be assumed to be present and must be treated.

(a) Give salbutamol (5 ml of salbutamol mixed with 3 ml of saline) by nebuliser or intermittent positive pressure respiration over 3 min up to four times each day.

(b) Aminophylline i.v. 5 mg/kg initially and then 0.5 mg/kg per hour thereafter. As well as being a bronchodilator, aminophylline may increase the force of diaphragmatic contraction. The dose may need adjusting in old or very ill patients (see p. 77).

(c) Steroids may also be given (e.g. hydrocortisone 200 mg 4-hourly) although the efficacy of these is arguable.

(4) Oxygen therapy.[5] Oxygen should be given in sufficient concentration to raise the Pa_{O_2} to at least 45 mmHg (6.0 kPa) and preferably 55 mmHg (7.3 kPa). To aim higher than this is unnecessary and, in view of the potential danger of oxygen therapy in this type of ventilatory failure, undesirable.

The danger of oxygen therapy arises because patients with a chronically raised Pa_{CO_2} rely not only on a rise in Pa_{CO_2}, as normal, but on a fall in Pa_{O_2} to stimulate respiration—the so-called hypoxic drive.[4] A sudden rise in Pa_{O_2} may reduce this hypoxic drive, and thus depress ventilation. This causes a further rise in Pa_{CO_2}, and may precipitate CO_2 narcosis.

So, after you have measured arterial blood gases, start with the 24% oxygen mask. Measure the arterial gases again after 1 h.

(i) If the Pa_{O_2} is above 55 mmHg (7.3 kPa); and Pa_{CO_2} has not gone up by more than 10 mmHg (1.3 kPa), continue using 24% O_2.

(ii) If the Pa_{O_2} is below 55 mmHg (7.3 kPa) and the Pa_{CO_2} has not gone up more than 10 mmHg (1.3 kPa), progress to 28% O_2 by Ventimask (4 l/min). Measure the Pa_{CO_2} again in a further hour and if situation (ii) still obtains, you may progress to the 35% Ventimask (8 l/min).

(iii) If the Pa_{CO_2} has risen more than 10 mmHg (1.3 kPa), you are in grave danger of inducing CO_2 narcosis. Do not increase (or lower) O_2 concentration but intensify all other aspects of treatment, particularly the conjunction of physiotherapy and respiratory stimulants. If the Pa_{CO_2} goes on rising despite this, you will have to decide if intermittent positive pressure respiration (IPPR) should be used. This can be a difficult decision, and depends particularly on the usual respiratory status of your patient. If he is a respiratory cripple, then IPPR is unlikely to be of lasting benefit and you may have difficulty weaning him off the ventilator.

(iv) Occasionally, patients are given high O_2 concentration by mistake, or in ignorance. This may lead to the rapid development of CO_2 narcosis. It is always best to assume that deterioration in the condition of a patient with ventilatory and hypoxaemic failure is due to CO_2 narcosis. Faced with this deteriorating situation:

(a) do not immediately increase the inspired O_2 concentration;
(b) prevent anybody else from doing so;
(c) measure the blood gases;
(d) if the chest signs have changed, repeat the chest x-ray to exclude pneumothorax or massive pulmonary collapse;
(e) intensify physiotherapy;
(f) if the Pao_2 is above 55 mmHg (7.3 kPa) and the $Paco_2$ either above 90 mmHg (12 kPa) or has risen by more than 10 mmHg (1.3 kPa) from your initial reading, reduce the O_2 to 24% by Ventimask, and use a respiratory stimulant;
(g) if the Pao_2 is below 35 mmHg (4.7 kPa) as well as $Paco_2$ being high, give a respiratory stimulant without altering the O_2 until the $Paco_2$ has improved;
(h) keep measuring the blood gases; you may have to consider IPPR if things go on deteriorating.

(5) Respiratory stimulants. These are used to:

(i)   wake up the patient and help him to cooperate,
(ii) counteract CO_2 narcosis (as above),
(iii) counteract respiratory depression.

Remember, in this context, that you must not sedate patients in respiratory failure. In fact, always write **NO NIGHT SEDATION** on their charts, so that no-one else sedates them either!

The best drug to use is doxapram, in a dose of 1.5 mg/min, increasing by 0.5 mg/min at ½-hourly intervals if there has been no improvement to a maximum of 3.0 mg/min.

Ethamivan 5% 2.5 ml i.v. may also be used, as may nikethamide 2–5 ml (0.5–1.25 mg) i.v. repeated ½-hourly as necessary.

If respiratory depression is due to opiates, naloxone, which is a specific opiate antagonist, can be used in doses of 0.4 mg given i.v. over 3 min. This may be repeated to a total dose of 1.2 mg. As it has a shorter duration of action than the opiates, it may need to be repeated.

(6) Heart failure. The measures outlined above result in a substantial diuresis. However, in the presence of gross or persistent CCF the following measures can be employed.

(i) Diuretics.

(ii) Digoxin, particularly if the patient has uncontrolled atrial fibrillation. Patients in respiratory failure have an enhanced sensitivity to digoxin, which is therefore best not used unless there is atrial fibrillation.

(iii) Do not forget that weight is a useful indicator of fluid balance—so weigh your patient daily.

(iv) In polycythaemic patients, diuresis may cause increased sludging of blood, and precipitate thrombosis. This may be prevented by venesection of 3 units of blood, and replacement with an equal amount of Haemaccel or dextran 70. This in itself may be sufficient to improve renal blood flow and initiate a diuresis; we consider this mode of therapy to be desirable in men with a PCV >54, and women >50.

PURE VENTILATORY FAILURE

(1) There are occasions when the underlying problem is rapidly reversible, e.g. administration of naloxone to persons with opiate-induced respiratory depression (see above).

(2) If no such specific therapy is available, the initial decision is when to institute artificial respiration.

(3) To make a decision you have to make appropriate measurements.

(i) Minute volume (measured with a Wright spirometer). If this is over 4 l/min the patient is very unlikely to require artificial ventilation.

(ii) Vital capacity (measured with a portable, bedside vitalograph). If the vital capacity remains above 1.5 litres, artificial ventilation will probably be unnecessary. The vital capacity should be measured at least daily in patients with progressive neurological lesions.

(iii) The blood gases should be measured if there is any doubt about the patient's respiratory status. If the $P\text{aCO}_2$ is raised, artificial ventilation should be instituted.

(4) Physiotherapy should be given routinely to help prevent sputum retention and infection.

(5) In unconscious patients without a gag reflex, or patients whose disease affects swallowing as well as breathing, inhalation of secretion or vomit must be prevented by passing an endotracheal tube.

(6) All this should be done in conjunction with the anaesthetists.

HYPOXAEMIC FAILURE

Treatment of the underlying disease should, of course, be initiated.

(1) Oxygen may be given by an MC mask (which delivers a concentration of 50–60% to the mouth, if the flow rate is 6 l/min) as there is no risk of CO_2 narcosis. However, be sure not to raise the PaO$_2$ too high (above 100 mmHg (13.3 kPa)) because high O_2 concentration can be damaging to lung tissue.

(2) Artificial ventilation should be resorted to if the PaO$_2$ cannot be maintained above about 50 mmHg (6.7 kPa), or if the effort of breathing is becoming intolerable.

REFERENCES

General

Crofton J., Douglas A. (1975). *Respiratory Disease*, 2nd edn. Oxford: Blackwell Scientific.
Hunter A. R. (1972). *Essentials of Artificial Ventilation of the Lungs*. London: Churchill Livingstone.

Respiratory failure

1   Clark T. J. H. (1972). Respiratory failure. *Br. J. Hosp. Med.*; **7:** 692.
2   Flenley D. C. (1978). Clinical hypoxia—causes, consequences and correction. *Lancet*; **i:** 542.
3   Howard P. (1983). Drugs or oxygen for hypoxic cor pulmonale. *Br. Med. J.*; **287:** 1159.
4   Leitch A. G. (1981). The hypoxic drive to breathing in man. *Lancet*; **i:** 428.
5   Woo S. W., Hedley Whyte J. (1973). Oxygen therapy—the titration of a potentially dangerous drug. *Br. J. Hosp. Med.*; **9:** 487.

Severe attacks of asthma[4]

DIAGNOSIS

(1) Recurrent reversible attacks of wheezing are the hallmarks of asthma, and if despite treatment such an attack lasts for more than 6 h, this is a serious situation with a real risk of unexpected death.[1]

(2) Pulmonary oedema may cause wheezing and mimic asthma quite closely (see p. 40), but other causes of dyspnoea (see p. 335) are usually easily differentiated from asthma.

(3) An attack is usually precipitated by a combination of factors, which include infection, allergy and emotion.

(4) Severe attacks are characterised by the following.

   (i)   The patient who is too breathless to speak.

   (ii)   Tachycardia of more than 120 beats/min.

   (iii) Pulsus paradoxus.[6] In acute asthmatic attacks paradox is usually, but not invariably, present. When it is present the degree of paradox reflects the degree of airways obstruction. In a severe attack the difference in systolic arterial pressure between inspiration and expiration may be as much as 100 mmHg (13.3 kPa), the normal difference being not more than 5 mmHg (0.7 kPa).

   (iv)   A 'silent' chest. There is insufficient air being moved to cause a wheeze.

   (v)   Cyanosis.

   (vi)   Hypercapnia. Figure 21 demonstrates that in most cases of asthma, the $P\text{aco}_2$ is low, and that a patient with a high $P\text{aco}_2$ is mortally ill. Some authorities suggest that any asthmatic who has a $P\text{aco}_2$ above 50 mmHg (6.7 kPa) when first seen should be ventilated forthwith, but in most circumstances it is reasonable to undertake management as outlined below.

   (vii) A respiratory rate above 30/min.

   (viii) A peak expiratory flow rate (PEFR) <100 l/min.

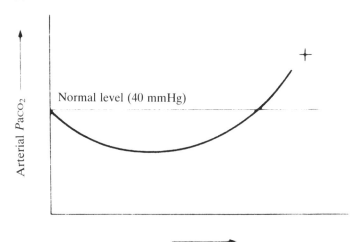

Fig. 21 Relationship between the Pa_{CO_2} and the severity of the asthmatic attack.

MANAGEMENT

Measurements of pulse rate, respiratory rate, degree of paradox and arterial blood gases are mandatory. So is an initial chest x-ray, as a pneumothorax (see p. 80) or massive pulmonary collapse (see p. 84) may complicate an asthmatic attack, and require treatment in its own right. Peak expiratory flow rate and, if you have a spirometer, forced expiratory volume in 1 s (FEV_1) are essential baseline measurements, changes of which provide a simple way of assessing progress.

Put up a drip and then treat the following aspects as described.

(1)
    The wheezing.

    (i)   Hydrocortisone in an initial dose of 4 mg/kg i.v. stat. and 3–4 mg/kg i.v. 6-hourly thereafter until the patient is better.[8] Oral prednisone 40 mg/day should be started at the same time, as corticosteroids may take 6–8 h to take effect.[5]

(ii)   Salbutamol is best given as an aerosol via a respirator:
       1–2 ml of 0.5% salbutamol respirator solution contain
       5–10 mg of salbutamol, and should be given on two occa-
       sions about 1 h apart. If, on the basis of PEFR, there is no
       improvement, you should try one of the other bron-
       chodilators mentioned below, as well as continuing sal-
       butamol 4-hourly. Salbutamol may also be given i.v.,
       starting at a dose of 5 μg/min and increasing to 20 μg/min
       as necessary.

(iii) Aminophylline should be given at a loading dose of
       5 mg/kg infused over 30 min, and 0.5 mg/kg each hour
       thereafter, aiming to obtain a serum level between 8 mg/l
       and 20 mg/l. Plasma levels should be checked at 24 h, and
       if your patient has CCF, liver disease or is taking oral
       theophylline, the above recommended doses should be
       halved.[3,7]

(iv)   Adrenaline and isoprenaline should be avoided unless
       you can be certain that your patient has not been using an
       aerosol, in which case give adrenaline 1 : 1000 0.5 ml
       subcutaneously.

(v)   Ipratropium bromide, an inhaled atropine-like com-
       pound, causes bronchodilatation by blocking vagal
       reflexes, and has an additive effect with salbutamol. Give
       250–500 μg in 4 ml of saline solution by nebulisers on
       two occasions, 1 h apart.[9]

(vi)   It makes good pharmacological sense to alternate nebul-
       ised salbutamol and ipratropium bromide, giving one or
       other initially at hourly, and then at 2-hourly intervals.
       This may pose logistic problems, but is an ideal to strive
       towards.

(2) Hypoxia. Start by giving 40% O_2 via a Ventimask until you
    know the blood gases. If the Pa_{CO_2} is raised, indicating that the
    patient's condition is critical, give O_2 as suggested on page 71,
    but bear in mind that ventilatory support will almost certainly
    be required in this group of patients. If the Pa_{CO_2} is below
    40 mmHg (5.3 kPa), you can give any concentration of O_2
    necessary to raise the Pa_{O_2} to 80 mmHg (10.7 kPa).

(3) Distress. A severe asthmatic attack is alarming for all con-
    cerned. However, you must not resort to sedation to allay the
    anxiety of your patient; rely on massive and repeated verbal
    reassurance. Try and exude confidence (which you will be far

from feeling). Your patient's distress is entirely justified. He will be relieved as soon as he begins to get better; if he deteriorates, hypnotics only make matters worse.

(4) Infection. Recent trials have questioned the routine use of antibiotics in acute asthma.[2] However, we feel their use is usually justified, so give either amoxycillin (250 mg i.v. 6-hourly) or oral tetracycline (500 mg q.d.s.) or cotrimoxazole (tabs. ii b.d.).

(5) Dehydration. Should be assumed to be present and should be corrected with adequate i.v. fluid (1.5 l of 5% dextrose and 500 ml of 0.9% saline (154 mmol/l) in the first 24 h is a reasonable amount, although up to 6 l of fluid may be needed). Correction of dehydration helps make the sputum less tenacious.

(6) Allergy. Removing the patient to hospital often removes him from the allergen. Clearly he must be prevented from coming into contact with any allergens to which he has a known sensitivity.

(7) Acidosis. Correction with appropriate amounts of $NaHCO_3$ as calculated from the base deficit (see p. 302) can give rise to considerable improvement.

(8) Hypokalaemia. This often occurs in acute asthma, and potassium supplements should be added to the i.v. solutions as necessary.

(9) Inspissated plugs of sputum. These are present in the airways of most severe asthmatics. Physiotherapy is not likely to shift them, and is both impractical and undesirable in the acute attack. As mentioned in (5) above, hydration is helpful in shifting these plugs.

(10) Deterioration of clinical condition and arterial blood gases. If your patient's clinical condition and arterial blood gases deteriorate despite the above measures, then ventilation with a powerful volume cycled respiratory (IPPV) may well be necessary. In our experience, ventilation is rarely necessary, and only some 0.3% of patients in status require this support. It is important to have a drip up, preferably with a CVP line, before IPPV is instituted, as hypovolaemia may be unmasked by IPPV. Take the arterial pressure, pulse and CVP at 10 min intervals and increase the infusion rate if necessary. This should be carried out in conjunction with your anaesthetic colleagues, and may be combined with bronchial lavage (see overleaf).

(11) Bronchial lavage. Like ventilation this is only rarely required, but if it is needed, it should be carried out via a fibreoptic bronchoscope down an endotracheal tube.

REFERENCES

1   Benatar S. R. (1986). Fatal asthma. *N. Engl. J. Med.*; **314:** 423.
2   Graham V. A. L. *et al.* (1982). Routine antibiotics in hospital management of acute asthma. *Lancet*; **i:** 418.
3   Leader (1983). Theophylline benefits and difficulties. *Lancet*; **i:** 607.
4   Leader (1986). Acute asthma. *Lancet*; **i:** 131.
5   Littenberg B., Gluck E. H. (1986). A controlled trial of methylprednisolone in the emergency treatment of acute asthma. *N. Engl. J. Med.*; **314**(3): 150.
6   McGregor M. (1979). Pulsus paradoxus. *N. Engl. J. Med.*; **301**(9): 478.
7   Powell J. R. *et al.* (1978). Theophylline disposition in acutely ill hospitalized patients. *Am. Rev. Resp. Dis.*; **118:** 229.
8   Rees J. (1984). Drug treatment in acute asthma. *Br. Med. J.*; **288:** 1747.
9   Ward M. J. *et al.* (1981). Ipratropium bromide in acute asthma. *Br. Med. J.*; **282:** 598.

Pneumothorax[2,3]

This is often due to the rupture of a subpleural bleb in an otherwise fit person, usually a young adult male. It may also complicate other respiratory conditions, such as asthma, chronic bronchitis or emphysema.

DIAGNOSIS

(1) In a fit person:

    (i) symptoms may be confined to slight dyspnoea or pleural pain, even when one lung is wholly collapsed;

    (ii) the signs are in combination diagnostic:

        (a) decreased movement on the affected side (not always present);

        (b) displacement of the trachea and apex beat away from the affected side (indicating mediastinal shift) may be present or absent, depending on the pressure in the pneumothorax;

        (c) increased resonance on the affected side (not always easy to detect);

        (d) distant breath sounds on the affected side (a good sign);

        (e) sometimes additional and often bizarre sounds may be heard—clicks or rubs.

(2) However, the history, symptoms and signs may be absent or may be thought to have an alternative explanation in patients who have other lung disease, such as emphysema or asthma. These patients may already be familiar from their previous episodes of infection or reversible airways obstruction, which look exactly similar. Their breath sounds may be difficult to hear at the best of times and a small pneumothorax may be impossible to detect. As they have no respiratory reserve and a missed diagnosis may be disastrous, they must always have a chest x-ray at each presentation.

(3) A pneumothorax is easier to see on a chest x-ray taken in expiration.

MANAGEMENT

If the patient is not breathless, has no associated lung disease and has a shallow pneumothorax (<30% reduction in lung volume on x-ray), it is reasonable to allow the air to resorb spontaneously. Otherwise, mechanical removal of the air is required. Traditionally, we have used a chest drain with an underwater seal to effect the removal of air. Recently, simple aspiration with a cannula has been used, and seems to be effective, less painful and associated with a shorter stay in hospital. Both methods are described below.

Simple aspiration[1]

We believe this to be the method of choice in patients with unilateral pneumothorax and without associated lung disease.

(1) Insert a 16-gauge i.v. Medicut into the pleural space, using local anaesthesia. Withdraw the needle, and connect the remaining plastic cannula through a three-way tap to a 60 ml syringe. The third outlet of your tap should be connected to a length of rubber tubing, the other end of which is placed in a jug of sterile water.

(2) Aspirate the air gently, 60 ml at a time, and expel it through the water.

(3) When you feel resistance on the aspirating syringe (probably due to re-expanded lung impinging against your cannula), or you have aspirated 2 l of air, stop your aspiration, and take a chest x-ray.

(4) If the lung is re-expanded, or you are left with a shallow (<30% volume) pneumothorax, merely observe your patient for 24 h, and take an x-ray after this. If the situation is unchanged or improving, no further intervention is required.

(5) If on either of the occasions outlined in (4) above, there is a persisting large pneumothorax, insert an intercostal drain.

Intercostal drain

(1) An intercostal drainage tube should therefore be inserted:

    (i)   if simple aspiration fails;

    (ii)   in any patient who has coexistent lung disease;

    (iii) in the presence of, or where there is history of, pneumothorax on the other side.

(2) The management of the intercostal drainage tube. The site of
choice for insertion of the intercostal tube is in the midaxillary
line in the fourth or fifth intercostal space. The midclavicular
line in the second intercostal space is a poor alternative because
sucking chest wounds have been known to occur after withdrawal of the tube and it leaves an unsightly scar. To enable a
problem-free insertion, we recommend blunt dissection of the
chest wall, preferring this to macho heavies leaning all their
weight on the tube, with the risk of spearing the patient to the
bed! The tube is attached to an underwater seal, e.g. a
thoracotomy drainage bottle with 100 m of sterile water in it,
the tip being directed up to the apex. Check the position on
chest x-ray. Make the patient cough a few times every hour to
allow the air to escape from the chest.

If the level in the underwater tube stops swinging, it is due to
one of the following.

(i)   The lung has re-expanded and is blocking off the end of
the tube. In this case clip off the tube, re-x-ray 24 h later
and if the lung has not gone down, remove the tube. If the
lung has gone down again, continue to drain until the lung
re-expands, then clip off, re-x-ray, etc.

(ii)   The holes in the tube may be occluded by chest wall or
partially re-expanded lung. Withdraw slightly and rotate.

(iii) The tube is blocked and it needs 'milking'. If this does not
unblock the tube, try to suck the tube free with a 50 ml
syringe. If this does not work, flush the tube out by
introducing 50 ml of sterile water into the chest. Finally,
change the tube.

If the lung does not expand even though the tube is patent,
attach the outlet tube of the thoracotomy bottle to gentle
suction (5–10 cmH$_2$O). Obviously the level will stop swinging.
Take the tube off suction every hour to check that the tube is
not blocked.

If, despite insertion of an intercostal tube and application of
suction, the lung still does not expand, consider bronchoscopy.
This may clear the main airways of sputum and allow air to
enter whilst the lung re-expands.

If an air leak either persists or recurs:

(a) check the connection of the intercostal tube to the
drainage bottle;

(b) seal the entry site of the intercostal tube in the chest by packing it with Tulle-gras to form an airtight dressing;

(c) increase the suction pressure to 10–15 cmH$_2$O if the leak is very free. If the air leak continues, there is probably a patent bleb on the lung surface. This will probably seal off in 36–48 h. Keep the tube on suction until the leak stops. Suck for a further 12 h, take off suction and watch the level in the underwater tube. If the chest maintains a negative pressure, i.e. the fluid level in the tube remains above the fluid level in the bottle, all is well. Clip off and re-x-ray in 24 h. If the lung is still expanded, take the tube out. If the two levels approximate and air begins to escape again, recommence suction and seek the advice of a thoracic surgical unit.

(3) Do not allow the thoracotomy bottle to be moved off the floor. If it is put on the bed locker, the contents will pass from the bottle into the chest. Keep two Spencer Wells clips on the thoracotomy bottle, and clip the tube off whenever you want to move the bottle or the patient.

(4) Physiotherapy should be routine for all patients with pneumothorax in an attempt to prevent sputum retention occurring. Remember to give any necessary pain relief prior to physiotherapy.[2]

(5) Pain control: both the illness and its treatment are painful. Give opiate analgesia as necessary, measuring arterial gases if there is any possibility of CO$_2$ retention (see p. 71).

(6) If the diagnosis of the pneumothorax has been delayed (>5 days), try simple aspiration first, as brisk re-expansion carries the risk of inducing unilateral pulmonary oedema.[4]

REFERENCES

1 Archer G. J. *et al.* (1985). Results of simple aspiration of pneumothoraces. *Br. J. Dis. Chest*; **79:** 177.

2 Crompton G. K. (1982). Spontaneous pneumothorax. *Hosp. Update*; 251.

3 Hart J. G. *et al.* (1983). Spontaneous pneumothorax in Norfolk. *Br. J. Dis. Chest*; **77:** 164.

4 Henderson A. F. (1985). Re-expansion pulmonary oedema: a potentially serious complication of delayed diagnosis of pneumothorax. *Br. Med. J.*; **291:** 593.

Massive pulmonary collapse

This is the term used to describe the complete collapse of a lobe or a lung. It may occur, of course, due to a spontaneous pneumothorax or following a chest injury with a sucking chest wound. The following remarks are confined to the absorption collapse which follows occlusion of one of the main airways.

DIAGNOSIS

(1) It may present itself as:

    (i)   sudden shortness of breath, with or without chest pain;
    (ii)   sudden worsening of an episode of acute infective bronchitis or asthma;
    (iii) fever, tachypnoea and tachycardia in an already ill patient, e.g. after major surgery;
    (iv) mental confusion.

(2) The signs are usually obvious. There is diminished movement on the affected side. The mediastinum is displaced towards the side of collapse, as demonstrated by shifting of the trachea and apex beat. There is dullness to percussion. If the major bronchi are obstructed, the breath sounds are diminished and there are usually no crackles. However, if the major bronchi remain patent but the peripheral bronchi are obstructed, the signs are those of consolidation, i.e. bronchial breathing, crackles and increased conduction of the spoken and whispered voice.

It is most commonly caused by:

(i)   a tenacious plug of sputum;
(ii)   a foreign body which may be radio-opaque, e.g. classically a fragment of tooth after dental anaesthesia;
(iii) carcinoma;
(iv) extrinsic pressure on the bronchus, e.g. hilar glands, aortic aneurysm, etc;
(v)   the endotracheal tube, at intubation performed for any reason, being inserted into one of the main bronchi, thus causing collapse of the other lung. This is an occasional cause.

MANAGEMENT

(1) If the diagnosis is suspected, a chest x-ray postero-anterior
(PA) and the appropriate lateral film should be taken. This will
demonstrate the volume of lung collapsed, possibly also a
foreign body in the trachea or bronchi, or malposition of an
endotracheal tube.

(2) Management is directed towards removal of obstruction and
obviously depends on the cause (see above). The following are
the two most common causes.

> (i) *Sputum.* If the patient is severely hypoxaemic or comat-
> ose, as, for example, after an operation, bronchoscopy
> should be undertaken immediately. Apart from this con-
> tingency there should be time to measure the arterial
> blood gases, and to assess the effects of vigorous
> physiotherapy with chest percussion and coughing. If this
> fails to produce an improvement within a few hours (as
> judged by a second chest x-ray), bronchoscopy should be
> undertaken. The timing will depend on the clinical state
> and the blood gases.
>
> (ii) *Foreign body.* Removal through a bronchoscope (usually
> a rigid one) should be undertaken without delay.

Other causes are less common and, as they are not usually amenable to urgent treatment, are outside the scope of this book.

Acute laryngeal obstruction

Acute laryngeal obstruction is a life-threatening emergency and if it is total and unrelieved, the patient will die in 3 min. Partial obstruction with stridor, cyanosis and a hoarse voice is dangerous and, if progressive, urgent treatment is necessary to prevent death. In total obstruction, speech is impossible. The diagnosis is usually clear from the history.

The cause is also fairly obvious.

(1) Trauma:
> strangulation,
> laceration,
> inhaled foreign bodies which, in adult practice, are usually a piece of food inhaled whilst the victim is eating,
> burns,
> irritant gases.

(2) Inflammatory:
> acute epiglottitis,[1]
> laryngotracheobronchitis.

(3) Diphtheria.

(4) Angioneurotic oedema.

(5) Tumours: laryngeal obstruction may occur as a primary presentation, or during radiotherapy to already diagnosed tumours.

It should not be confused with the obstruction caused by the tongue flopping back into the pharynx. This is of course easily relieved by lifting the jaw forward and inserting a pharyngeal airway.

MANAGEMENT

(1) Establish a better airway. Intubation may be difficult and occasionally impossible in these patients. So, once diagnosed, an experienced anaesthetist should be called urgently together with a surgeon proficient in tracheostomies.

(2) While awaiting their arrival, administer O_2 and obtain a tracheostomy set. Heliox (79% helium, 27% oxygen) mixture, if available, is more effective as the helium makes the mixture less viscous. It therefore effectively, albeit only temporarily, reduces stridor.

(3) If the patient continues to deteriorate with deepening cyanosis (despite vigorous respiratory efforts) and increasing pulse rate, and the anaesthetist has not yet arrived, an emergency tracheostomy should be performed.

This is a simple operation.

(i) Place the patient on his back with the neck extended.
(ii) Ask an assistant to hold the arms.
(iii) Steady the trachea between thumb and finger and slide a sharp knife between, preferably, the 3rd and 4th tracheal rings.
(iv) Rotate the blade through 90° to maintain an airway and insert tracheal dilators.

(4) In angioneurotic oedema or post-radiotherapy oedema, hydrocortisone i.v. 200 mg plus 0.5–1.0 ml 1 : 1000 adrenaline i.m. may reduce the obstruction sufficiently to avoid intubation.
(5) Patients with tumours and those undergoing a course of radiotherapy should be referred to the ENT surgeons immediately.
(6) The Heimlich manoeuvre.[2,3] If you are confronted with the problem of acute laryngeal obstruction from inhalation outside of the hospital environment (the café coronary syndrome), use of Heimlich's manoeuvre may be life saving.

The principle here is that a rapid upward thrust from below the xiphisternum pushes the diaphragm up, and forcefully expels air from the mouth. Any obstructing object is likewise forcefully and dramatically expelled.

The technique can be carried out in people sitting, standing or lying.

(i) Victim sitting or standing. The rescuer either stands or kneels behind the victim, encircling the victim's waist with one of his arms. With one hand, he makes a fist, and places his thumb slightly above the navel, and well below the tip of the xiphoid process, then covers the fist with his free hand, and presses into the victim's abdomen with a quick upward thrust. It may be necessary to repeat this thrust up to six times, although 60% of people are relieved of their obstruction after only two thrusts. The obstructing object may be expelled with such force as to hit a wall 3.7 m away, and should be identified whenever possible.

(ii) Victim lying. The victim is placed on his back, with hi
face looking directly forward. Facing the victim, th
rescuer kneels astride him. He puts the palm of one han
between the navel and xiphisternum, places the other o
top of it, and pushes upwards and inwards.

REFERENCES

1   Baker A. J. (1986). Adult epiglottitis. *N. Engl. J. Med.*; **314**
    1185.
2   Editorial (1975). Statement on the Heimlich manoeuvre. *J*
    Am. Med. Assoc.; **234:** 416.
3   Heimlich H. J. (1982). First aid for the choking child—bac
    blows and chest thrusts cause complications and death
    Paediatrics; **70:** 120.

Massive pleural effusions

DIAGNOSIS

(1) The patient usually has dyspnoea and may give a history of pleuritic pain.

(2) Differentiation from other causes of shortness of breath (see p. 335) is usually obvious on examination—the signs on the affected side being decreased movement, shift of the mediastinum to the opposite side, stony dullness, and decreased breath and voice sounds.

(3) The diagnosis is confirmed by a chest x-ray (see below).

MANAGEMENT

(1) The effusion must be aspirated if causing distress, whatever the cause.

(2) A chest x-ray—PA and the appropriate lateral—should be taken to determine the optimal site for aspiration and to delineate structures which must be avoided, such as the diaphragm. The diaphragm is attached to the sixth rib anteriorly, the seventh rib laterally and the ninth rib posteriorly. The sixth space laterally and eighth space posteriorly (tip of the scapula) are recommended aspiration sites.

(3) If you do not need to aspirate the effusion, withdrawing fluid via a 50 ml syringe is tedious and prolongs discomfort for the patient. Therefore, insert a needle into the chest in the normal way. Attach it to the wall suction (if you have it) via a sterile underwater seal as for a pneumothorax (see p. 82) and, by a gentle negative pressure (5–10 cmH$_2$O), aspirate fluid from the chest. If wall suction is not available, an evacuated sterile bottle can be used.[1]

(4) Stop aspirating if:

    (i)   1 litre is obtained;

    (ii)   the patient complains of central chest pain: this means mediastinal shift is beginning to occur and this can cause rapid cardiovascular collapse and the temptation to continue must be resisted;

(iii) the patient has a haemoptysis: this means that the lung surface has been pierced. It is not usually serious but is frightening for all concerned. Unless the needle has been advanced further than necessary, the lung has re-expanded sufficiently for aspiration to be stopped.

(5) If the effusions are bilateral, aspiration of the larger effusion is usually sufficient to relieve dyspnoea.

REFERENCE

1   Rutowska J. (1967). An easy method of aspiration for pleural effusions. *Hosp. Med.*; **2:** 370.

Adult respiratory distress syndrome (ARDS) (shock lung)[4,5,7]

DIAGNOSIS

(1) Shock lung is characterised by:

    (i)   tachypnoea;

    (ii) deteriorating $P_{a}O_2$;

    (iii) a decrease in lung compliance—usually to a level below 50 ml/cmH$_2$O;

    (iv) progressive diffuse infiltration on the chest x-ray, with associated widespread crackles, occurring in a patient who, within the preceding 48 h, has had an episode of hypotension.

(2) It is particularly likely to occur if the hypotensive episode was associated with:

    (i)   traumatised or dead tissue, as in crush injuries;

    (ii) circulating bacterial endotoxins, as in gram-negative septicaemia;

    (iii) fat emboli;

    (iv) amniotic fluid emboli;

    (v) intravascular haemolysis;

    (vi) difficult or lengthy surgery;

    (vii) primary lung conditions, such as severe infections, aspiration or contusion.

(3) It arises because of an increase in:

    (i)   pulmonary capillary permeability;

    (ii) pulmonary vascular resistance.

Both of these cause an increase in pulmonary interstitial fluid.

(4) It is associated with a normal PCWP initially. In shock lung, PCWP will be below 18 mmHg and is most reliably measured using a Swan–Ganz catheter (see p. 346) wedged in the lower half of the lung field. By contrast, in left ventricular failure, from which it must be distinguished, the PCWP is more than 25 mmHg, provided that the oncotic pressure is normal.

TREATMENT

Treatment is difficult, often prolonged, frequently unsuccessful and should be undertaken in association with your anaesthetic colleagues. It involves the following.

(1) Therapy directed toward the specific insult provoking shock lung.
(2) Early assisted ventilation. You should attempt to keep the P_{aO_2} around 70 mmHg (9.3 kPa) with added inspired O_2.[3] Early introduction of positive end expiratory pressure (PEEP) of up to 10 cmH$_2$O improves functional residual capacity, compliance, and thus oxygenation. Remember, however, that PEEP may drop the arterial pressure by decreasing left ventricular filling and this will be a limiting factor in its use.[1,6]

Indications for ventilation are as follows.

(i) A patient who is getting progressively more exhausted by the effort of breathing.
(ii) Respiratory rate of above 35/min.
(iii) P_{aO_2} of less than 70 mmHg (9.3 kPa) in spite of added O_2.[3]
(iv) Alveolar arterial oxygen differences (A-aDO$_2$) of greater than 50 mmHg (6.7 kPa).
The A-aDO$_2$ reflects the effective transfer of O_2 from the alveolus to the arterial blood. In a patient breathing room air with a P_{aO_2} of 150 mmHg (20 kPa):

$$\text{A-aDO}_2 = 150 - (P_{aO_2} + P_{aCO_2})\ 0.8$$

and is normally less than 20. (The value 0.8 in the above equation is the respiratory quotient.)
(v) Rising P_{aCO_2}. If the P_{aCO_2} is above 40 mmHg (5.3 kPa) you have left things too late.

(3) Careful fluid balance. The problem is that fluid replacement is a balancing act between keeping the filling pressure of the left ventricle high enough to sustain the cardiac output, and yet low enough to minimise transmembrane fluid flux into the lung.

(i) So which fluids should you use?

(a) Blood should be replaced if the hematocrit falls below 30%.

(b) Haemaccel or high molecular weight dextran (dextran 70) should be used to expand the plasma volume if necessary (see below).

(c) Crystalloid fluids should only be used sparingly to replace losses, as these fluids will, of course, tend to leak into the lung and aggravate the underlying problem.

(ii) How do you monitor replacement. This is difficult, for the following reasons.

(a) If your patient is ventilated with PEEP, central venous pressure (CVP) readings are unreliable.

(b) PCWP recordings only help to exclude coexistent left ventricular failure.

(c) Therefore, clinical judgement is of paramount importance. You should strive towards a patient with warm peripheries, good urinary output, clear mental faculties and a systolic arterial pressure above 90 mmHg, but, if in doubt, err on the side of keeping your patient 'dry' rather than 'wet'.

(4) Antibiotics. As infection does not seem to play an important role in the genesis of shock lung, only use antibiotics if there is purulent sputum.

(5) Corticosteroids. There is no evidence that these are helpful once shock lung has developed. Massive doses (2 g solumedrone i.v. each day for 2 days) may be helpful if inhalation of vomit has occurred.[9] If there is bronchospasm, hydrocortisone in the same doses as used for acute asthma (see p. 75) should be used.

(6) Correction of acidosis. A low pH increases capillary leakage. Cautious correction with $NaHCO_3$ (see p. 302), with due regard to Na^+ balance, should be attempted.

(7) Fluid balance. Likewise, a raised urea (above 15 mmol/l) increases capillary leakage; careful attention to fluid balance and nutrition will help forestall this problem.

(8) Correction of stress ulceration. In patients who are critically ill, acute gastrointestinal bleeding can be prevented by using enteral feeding wherever possible, and either cimetidine or antacids. Rational use of these agents is based on a severity index score of illness. Each of the problems outlined below gets a score of 1.

(i)   Documented respiratory insufficiency for 24 h.
(ii)   Circulatory collapse (BP persistently <90 mmHg or requiring pressor agents).
(iii)   Patients with documented sepsis.
(iv)   Patients with CCF, myocardial infarct or arrhythmias warranting therapy.
(v)   Creatinine level acutely raised to above 250 μmol/l.
(vi)   Patients with a Glasgow coma scale score <10.
(vii)   Patients on high-dose steroids.
(viii) Patients with a platelet count <50 000 or prothrombin time of less than 30% of the control.
(ix)   Bilirubin >90 μmol/l with or without hepatitis.

The maximum severity index score is 9. Carefully controlled trials suggest that in scores of 0–2, cimetidine 300 mg i.v. 6-hourly or antacids (Maalox) to keep the intragastric pH >4.0 (average 20 ml Maalox each 2 h) are equally effective, whereas for scores 3–6, Maalox is considerably more effective than cimetidine, and for scores above 6, prophylaxis is to no avail.

We suggest using prophylaxis along these lines.[2,8]

(9) Physiotherapy. Atelectasis occurs early in the shock lung syndrome. Encouraging regular sighing or deep respirations, making sure your patient coughs and is turned frequently, are vital therapeutic manoeuvres.

(10) Membrane oxygenation. A recent trial showed no increase in survival with this heroic mode of therapy.

REFERENCES

1   Harrison M. J. (1986). PEEP and CPAP. *Br. Med. J.*; **292:** 643.
2   Leader (1978). Gastro-intestinal bleeding in acute respiratory failure. *Br. Med. J.*; **1:** 531.
3   Leader (1981). Acute oxygen therapy. *Lancet*; **i:** 980.
4   Leader (1986). Adult respiratory distress syndrome. *Lancet*; **i:** 301.
5   Lloyd J. E. *et al.* (1984). Permeability pulmonary oedema. *Arch. Intern. Med.*; **144:** 143.
6   Rounds S., Brody J. S. (1984). Putting PEEP in perspective. *N. Engl. J. Med.*; **311:** 323.
7   Wallace P. G. M., Spence A. A. (1983). Adult respiratory distress syndrome. *Br. Med. J.*; **286:** 1167.

8   Zinner M. J. *et al.* (1981). The prevention of upper gastro-
     intestinal tract bleeding in patients in an I.T.U. *Surg. Gynaecol.
     Obstet.*; **153:** 214.
9   Zorab J. S. M. (1984). Pulmonary aspiration. *Br. Med. J.*; **222:**
     1631.

Pulmonary aspiration syndrome[1]

Aspiration of substances into the lungs can be divided into three categories.

(1) Aspiration of toxic materials. The significant fluids here are acids, alcohols, volatile hydrocarbons, oils and animal fats. These produce a chemical pneumonitis; the most important factor in the production of the pneumonitis is the acidity of the aspiration fluid—fluids with a pH below 2.5 consistently cause chemical damage. Postpartum aspiration pneumonitis (Mendelson's syndrome) is the classical example of this chemical pneumonitis.

(2) Aspiration of non-toxic materials—either liquids with a pH >7.3 or particulate matter. Here the damage relates to the composition and/or volume of the aspirated material. Chemical pneumonitis does not occur, although secondary bacterial infection may.

(3) Bacterial aspiration. This is characterised by the onset of a bacterial pneumonia 24 h or so after the inhalation of an inoculum of bacteria. Poor oral hygiene is the most frequent predisposing condition, and the resultant pneumonia is usually a result of a mixed bacterial infection, including anaerobes.

The remainder of this section refers solely to the chemical pneumonitis produced by toxic aspiration.

DIAGNOSIS

(1) There is usually a clear predisposing cause.

    (i)   Loss of airway protective reflexes, as in comatose, anaesthetised, heavily sedated or neurologically compromised patients.

    (ii)   Oesophageal disorders or decreased gastric emptying time increase the potential for aspiration.

    (iii) Iatrogenic factors, such as the presence of nasogastric tubes or tube feeding enhance the likelihood of aspiration.

(2) Chemical damage to the lungs produces bronchospasm and a massive exudation of fluid into the lungs. This causes dyspnoea, wheezing and a cough productive of frothy pink sputum. Hypoxia, hypotension, tachycardia and the adult respiratory distress syndrome may develop (see p. 91).

(3) Chest x-ray will show patchy alveolar infiltrates; the $Pa\text{CO}_2$ will be low or normal, $Pa\text{O}_2$ low.

MANAGEMENT

(1) Suction to clear the oropharynx of secretions should be undertaken immediately following aspiration. If the airway protective reflexes are thought to be compromised, your patient should be intubated.

(2) Oxygen therapy should be commenced with an MC mask to deliver 50% inspired O_2 concentration. Continuous positive airways pressure (CPAP) is helpful as it improves the balance between ventilation and perfusion. If you cannot maintain the $Pa\text{O}_2$ above 65 mmHg (8.6 kPa) consider mechanical ventilation.

(3) Bronchodilators should be used as for asthma (see p. 77) to control the wheezing. The role of steroids is controversial; we give one dose of solumedrone 2 g i.v., recognising that the efficacy of this is unproven.

(4) Antibiotics. Bacterial superinfection occurs within 72 h in about half of the patients with chemical pneumonitis. The infecting organisms are derived from the oropharynx, and so will be a mixed flora including anaerobes. The role of prophylactic antibiotics is unclear. In practice, we usually give metronidazole orally or rectally (see p. 311) and a penicillin (see p. 309).

(5) Fluids. Hypovolaemia, due in part to extravasation of fluids into the lungs, should be corrected. As in ARDS (see p. 91), the lung capillaries are leaky, so you have to achieve the delicate balance of a vascular volume sufficient to provide good perfusion with as low a left ventricular end-diastolic pressure as possible.

Remember that you should aim to prevent aspiration occurring. Always position patients with compromised airways in the semiprone position, and be prepared to intubate as necessary. Regular antacids or H_2 antagonists to raise the pH of gastric contents (see p. 109) are also advisable in those who are predisposed to aspirate.

REFERENCE

1   Vender J. S. (1986). Pulmonary aspiration. In *Update in Intensive Care and Emergency Medicine*, p. 71. New York: Springer Verlag.

Community-acquired severe pneumonia [1,3,5]

Pneumonia is often the terminal illness in the elderly and, as such, should be managed on its merits. Pneumonia can, however, occur in otherwise healthy adults. It may strike with extraordinary rapidity, and at its most severe, someone who appears well in the morning may be dead by evening. The pathology of this particularly cataclysmic, and happily uncommon, variant is usually staphylococcal superinfection of a lung already damaged by a viral pneumonitis. In Britain, the usual pathogen in the commoner less severe presentation is *Streptococcus pneumoniae* (75% of cases).[4] The next most common forms are those due to the so-called atypical pathogens—the main ones being *Mycoplasma* and *Legionella*. As indicated above, *Staphylococcus* is an uncommon cause, as are *Haemophilus influenzae* and *Klebsiella*. In some cases, a virus alone is thought to be responsible, frequently the influenza virus.

DIAGNOSIS

(1) There may have been a preceding viral illness, which, initially seeming trivial, may progress to dyspnoea, fever, cough productive of yellow and often bloodstained sputum and pleuritic pain. In the severest cases, there may be progression through mental confusion and disorientation to a state of septic shock with circulatory collapse. In these circumstances, admittedly only a small proportion of the whole, you may be presented with a hypoxic, cyanosed, disorientated, peripherally cool, hypotensive patient, and in this group mortality is high.

(2) The auscultatory signs are those of widespread, often asymmetrical areas of diminished breath sounds. There may also be focal evidence of consolidation, and an accompanying pleural rub. Chest x-ray may show lobar consolidation or non-specific diffuse lung shadowing.

MANAGEMENT

Take blood for arterial blood gases, full blood picture (FBP), including white cell count, electrolytes, urea and blood cultures. Also, save a specimen for viral antibodies. Do a CXR and ECG and send sputum for gram-staining and culture. Then treat the following as indicated.

(1) *Hypoxia.* Pa_{O_2} <60 mmHg (8.0 kPa) is the rule in this type of patient. Correction should be with a high concentration of O_2 by MC mask, unless there is evidence of chronic airflow obstruction. If the Pa_{O_2} persists below 60 mmHg (8.0 kPa) or the Pa_{CO_2} persists above 40 mmHg (5.3 kPa) on face mask oxygen, assisted ventilation will be required and you should consult with your anaesthetic colleagues.

(2) *Infection.* You will usually have to begin antibiotics before you know what the organism is.

    (i)   Most patients will turn out to have *Strep. pneumoniae*, and will respond to penicillin, so give benzyl penicillin 1.2 g i.v. 6-hourly.

    (ii)   If there is an atypical history—a disproportionate degree of systemic rather than respiratory symptoms—you should use erythromycin 500 mg 6-hourly. Likewise, if there has been no response to penicillin in 48 h, you should switch to erythromycin.

    (iii)   Some authorities suggest that all community-acquired pneumonias should receive both the above drugs from the start, and this is a not unreasonable approach.

    (iv)   If there has been a recent influenza outbreak, or there is cavitation on the CXR, you should treat for the staphylococci as well. Add flucloxacillin 500 mg to the penicillin.

    (v)   If the patient is desperately ill, consider adding either:

        (a) fucidin 500 mg i.v. 6-hourly, or

        (b) chloramphenicol 1.0 g 6-hourly i.v., which is the drug of choice for *H. influenzae* and is also effective against many staphylococci.

    (vi)   If there has been any question of inhalation, add metronidazole (see p. 311), as many of the inhaled bacteria will be anaerobes, and not all of these will be sensitive to penicillin.

(3) To help the patient cough up *infected sputum*, physiotherapy is often given. However, trials have shown it to be of no benefit.[2]

(4) *Circulatory collapse.* In the few patients who develop circulatory collapse, the prognosis is very grave. Conventional therapy involving fluid replacement under CVP control (see p. 343) should be instituted. The only practical difference is that we suggest using predominantly colloid rather than crystalloid infusion to support the circulation since the latter is more likely to extravasate into the already damaged lung. Insertion of a Swan–Ganz catheter, enabling you to measure pulmonary artery and pulmonary wedge pressure, will help you to manage fluid replacement in these patients. Exudation of fluid into the lungs of these patients is usually due to parenchymal lung damage. This may be clinically difficult to distinguish from left ventricular failure, but by measuring the PCWP with the Swan–Ganz catheter, you should be able to distinguish between the two (see p. 346).

The role of steroids is equivocal; we do not use them.

As always, if your patient is critically ill the care given by highly skilled nurses in an ITU is a critical factor in determining the outcome. You forget this at your patient's peril.

REFERENCES

1   Donowitz G. R., Mandell G. L. (1983). Empiric therapy for pneumonia. *Rev. Infect. Dis.* **5** (suppl.): 40.
2   Graham W. G., Bradley D. A. (1978). Efficacy of chest physiotherapy and intermittent positive pressure breathing in the resolution of pneumonia. *N. Engl. J. Med.*; **299:** 624.
3   Lockley M. R., Wise R. (1984). Pneumococcal infections. *Br. Med. J.*; **288:** 1179.
4   Macfarlane J. T. *et al.* (1982). Hospital study of adult community acquired pneumonia. *Lancet*; **ii:** 255.
5   Rees J. (1985). Respiratory infection. *Med. Educ. Int.*; p. 537.

Gastrointestinal

Massive upper gastrointestinal haemorrhage[8,17]

This presents itself in the ways listed below.

(1) Haematemesis and/or blood per rectum (melaena). Remember, however, that malaena alone may arise from anywhere in the GI tract down to and including the caecum.
(2) Cardiovascular collapse.
(3) Postural hypotension and fainting. A fall in systolic arterial pressure of greater than 10 mmHg on sitting the patient up indicates an acute blood loss in excess of 1000 ml.
(4) Symptoms of anaemia—fatigue, shortness of breath and angina—which, however, more often result from chronic blood loss.

It is usually caused by the following.

(1) Bleeding peptic ulcers (possibly drug induced, see (2) below).
(2) Acute gastric erosions.[9] These may:

    (i)   be drug induced (salicylate, steroids, phenylbutazone and indomethacin being common offenders);[4]
    (ii) occur after an alcoholic binge;
    (iii) occur in any patient seriously ill for whatever reason.

(3) Reflux oesophagitis, with or without hiatus hernia.
(4) The Mallory–Weiss syndrome[5] (traumatic oesophageal tear usually secondary to prolonged retching or vomiting).
(5) Bleeding oesophageal or gastric varices (look for evidence of liver disease).

It may occasionally be caused by:

(1) gastric neoplasm;
(2) coagulation disorder (look for bleeding elsewhere, including prolonged bleeding from puncture sites);
(3) connective tissue disease, such as Osler–Weber–Rendu syndrome (look for telangiectasia).

MANAGEMENT

Management of this emergency always requires close collaboration between surgeons and physicians and sometimes radiologists. Every case should be treated jointly, preferably in an intensive care unit, as follows.

(1) **Restoration and maintenance of circulating volume** and hence tissue perfusion. This is urgent if blood loss sufficient to cause poor peripheral perfusion has already occurred (see p. 295) or the patient has a systolic arterial pressure of below 90 mmHg and a pulse rate of above 100 beats/min. It is always necessary to take cases of GI blood loss seriously as patients may continue to bleed in hospital. Therefore, in all cases of major bleeding:

(i)   take blood for haemoglobin PCV electrolytes and urea, group and cross-match 2 l initially (and save the serum in case more blood becomes necessary), and kaolin–cephalin time, prothrombin time and platelet count; remember, haemoglobin concentration may be misleading before haemodilution occurs;

(ii)   set up a CVP line;

(iii) replace the circulating volume; two basic questions must be answered.

(a) *What with?*

—Compatible blood is clearly the fluid of choice, and should be available within a few hours.

—If the situation is not desperate, give 0.9% N saline (154 mmol/l) while waiting.

—However, if you consider that a colloid is necessary before compatible blood is available, give plasma, or dextran with an average molecular weight of 70 000.

Do not give doses in excess of 15 ml/kg per 24 h as they may cause disseminated intravascular coagulation. Do not forget to take blood for cross-matching before giving this. Haemaccel is a suitable alternative (see p. 299). The use of artificial blood may also increase with the increasing anxiety about AIDS (see p. 300).

—In desperate circumstances, 'O' negative blood may be given without cross-matching.

(b) *How much?*

—If you have a CVP line (which you should have), transfuse blood rapidly until the CVP rises into the upper half of the normal range (i.e. 1 cm above the manubriosternal joint with the patient supine, see p. 342). The patient will become warm and tranquil, and the arterial pressure and pulse will return to normal. If this does not happen, it implies the patient is continuing to bleed, and you must, therefore, continue to transfuse (while, of course, considering other possible therapeutic manoeuvres).

If, after your initial resuscitation has been successful, the CVP drops suddenly (i.e. a fall of greater than 5 cmH$_2$O in less than 2 h, this should be taken as an indication of re-bleeding. Further indications, such as a fresh haematemesis or fresh blood up the nasogastric tube, a fall in arterial pressure, or restlessness and sweating, may then develop. All these will alert you to the need for further blood and action.

—If you have no CVP measurements, transfuse the patient until he is warm, tranquil and has a restored arterial pressure and pulse rate. A rate of about 0.6 litres (1 pint) of blood/h is reasonable to start with.

—In all cases, look for the usual clinical signs of overload (raised JVP, crepitus at the lung bases, oedema). If these occur, slow down the infusion rate and give a diuretic, e.g. frusemide 40 mg i.v. and ouabain (see p. 16).

(iv) Consider passing a nasogastric tube. This has the advantage that:

(a) it rids the stomach of Guinness, pills and blood;
(b) it may be useful in diagnosing re-bleeding;
(c) it may be helpful to know the pH of the stomach contents, so the appropriate dose of antacids or cimetidine can be given;
(d) the stomach can be emptied prior to endoscopy.

However:

(a) it is uncomfortable and sometimes distressing for the patient;
(b) it may cause further bleeding;
(c) its use is associated with an increase in respiratory complications.

The authors do not use it routinely.

(v)   In some patients, particularly the elderly who have had gradual blood loss, it is wise to give frusemide from the onset of the transfusion, as heart failure develops easily in this group.

(2) **Determining the cause**. This is undertaken when initial resuscitation is underway, and may be suggested by the patient's history and by examination. In around 30% of patients, no cause will be found, despite careful evaluation.

Further investigations are as follows:

(i)   Endoscopy, which we usually carry out within 24 h of the patient's admission.[12,16] Although the site of bleeding will be visualised in most cases, giving comfort to physician and patient alike, early routine endoscopy has not altered the outlook in upper GI haemorrhage. However, now that endoscopic evidence of a blood vessel in an ulcer base is recognised to be associated with a high incidence of re-bleeding, and thus with the need for early surgery, the full value of endoscopy may be greater than we presently realise.[17] It is anyway worth remembering that patients with liver disease may bleed from peptic ulcers as well as from varices, and actually seeing the bleeding site will sort out this problem for you.

(ii) If the patient continues to bleed rapidly after admission, the stomach is likely to be full of blood, and endoscopy unrewarding. In these circumstances arteriography gives a high degree of diagnostic accuracy, and is probably the investigation of choice.[1] It takes only ½ h and can be done while a theatre is being prepared, if the surgeons consider operation is necessary. Arteriography may also be an invaluable therapeutic technique (p. 112).

(iii) Emergency barium or Gastrografin meals may be helpful in the diagnosis of upper GI bleeding (particularly where endoscopy is not available). Consult with the radiologist as soon as practical.

(3) **Stopping the bleeding.**

General measures

(i)   Tranexamic acid 1 g 6-hourly i.v. for 48 h, and then 500 mg 6-hourly, has been found to reduce mortality i upper GI bleeding, though not the frequency of recurrent haemorrhage or surgery. Until the situation is clarified, we do not advocate its routine use.[2]

(ii) Somatostatin, a potent inhibitor of acid and pepsin secretion by the stomach, is being evaluated. Infused at a rate of 250 µg/h for 72 h, it seems to confer some benefit, but should not yet be used routinely.[15]

Specific sites

- Peptic ulcer

    (i)   Cimetidine. A recent controlled trial showed no benefit from this drug so far as prevention of re-bleeding is concerned.[2,8]

    (ii) Surgery undertaken to control bleeding may be considered if:

        (a) the patient continues to bleed for 12 h after admission;
        (b) the bleeding recurs in hospital;
        (c) the patient is over 50;
        (d) there is a previous history of bleeding, or a long history of ulcer trouble;
        (e) there is coexistence of another complication (e.g. perforation);
        (f) there is no more blood available;
        (g) perhaps most importantly, the endoscopist sees a vessel in the ulcer base.[3,17]

        There are some proponents of aggressive early surgery in the over-60s. This may certainly be one way of reducing the unacceptably high mortality.[13]

    (iii) Laser coagulation of a visible vessel in an ulcer base is an attractive therapeutic option for those with this facility.[10,18]

- Acute gastric erosions[9]

    (i)   Surgery should be avoided if possible as the condition is usually self-limiting.

    (ii) Cimetidine, 100 mg i.v./h in 5% dextrose should be infused, with the aim of maintaining the pH of the stomach contents above 5.

    (iii) Antacids. The best tested method of raising the pH of

stomach contents is by instilling 30 ml of antacid (e.g. Maalox) hourly into the stomach. This may have advantages over cimetidine.

- Oesophageal or gastric varices[7,11,19]

    (i)   Give vasopressin 20 units i.v. in 100 ml of 5% dextrose over 10 min. This substance lowers the portal venous pressure, and an effective dose causes pallor, colicky abdominal pain and evacuation of the bowel. It also causes coronary artery vasoconstriction, and should be used with caution in patients with ischaemic heart disease. The effect lasts about 45 min and the dose may be repeated 4-hourly,

    If it is available, use the new analogue of vasopressin, triglycyl lysine vasopressin. This has a longer half-life than vasopressin, causes fewer side-effects, and is more effective.[6] Give 2 mg by bolus i.v. injection 6-hourly. If bleeding persists, this dose may be doubled.

    (ii) If facilities for arteriography are available, the vasopressin is best given directly into the coeliac axis (at a dose of 0.2–0.7 units/min for 20 min.[1]

    (iii) If vasopressin fails, the Boyce modification of the Sengstaken Blakemore tube may be used.[14] A new tube should be used on each occasion; the upper GI tract should be aspirated via a nasogastric tube, and the bed-head should be elevated 15–20.5 cm (6–10 in). Spray the pharynx with 2% lignocaine; test the balloons for leaks; make sure which tube connects with which balloon, and, with the patient in a left lateral position, pass the well-lubricated tube into the stomach, either through the nose or the mouth. You may have to use a flexible wire to stiffen the tube if you have problems passing it. Fill the stomach balloon with about 100–150 cm^3 of radio-opaque dye to localise it (20 ml of 20% diodone in 100 ml of water) and inflate the oesophageal balloon to a pressure of 30 mmHg. The oesophageal balloon must not be inflated until the tube has been stabilised by the stomach balloon. Similarly, the nursing staff must be told that they must always deflate the oesophageal balloon before emptying the stomach balloon, otherwise the oesophageal balloon may ride up the oesophagus and obstruct the pharynx. With the stomach tube pulled firmly up against the oesophagogastric junction, tape it either to the patient or, preferably, a preformed traction pad.[14]

Both during insertion and when the tube is finally in place, constant low pressure (5 mmHg) suction should be applied to the accessory tube, which aspirates secretions from the oesophagus and hypopharynx; this ensures that the oesophagus is kept free from potentially dangerous secretions. Both balloons are left in place for 24–48 h, as necessary, then the oesophageal balloon is deflated. Some authorities recommend deflating the oesophageal balloon for 10 min every 6 h in the hope of minimising the occurrence of oesophageal necrosis. The tube is left in position another 24 h with the stomach balloon still full in case of re-bleeding. It is then removed (after emptying the stomach balloon!). No food or drink is allowed while the tube is in place, though drugs may be given via the stomach tube.

If used with care, the Sengstaken Blakemore tube will control oesophageal variceal bleeding in 90% of cases.[15]

The volumes of air and water mentioned above relate only to the Boyce modification of the Sengstaken tube; other varieties have different specifications and you should check this before using your tube.

(iv)   In view of the ineffectiveness of any shunting procedures to control bleeding, local injection of sclerosing agents into the varix (through a rigid or flexible gastroscope) is being tried—preliminary results are encouraging.[11]

(v)   Percutaneous transhepatic portal vein catheterisation with subsequent selective injection of gel-foam into the major venous supply of the varices (left gastric and short gastric veins) is a promising new technique.

(vi)   Emergency transection of the oesophagus is still an occasional life saver, particularly if the 'gun' technique is used to staple the oesophagus.[7]

- Oesophageal bleeding due either to reflux oesophagitis or the Mallory–Weiss syndrome

(i)   Medical measures usually suffice, but if bleeding persists, surgery may become necessary.

(ii)   Local arterial perfusion with vasopressin 0.2–0.4 i.u/min for up to 36 h may give temporary or sometimes permanent relief.[1]

(4) **Arteriography as a therapeutic manoeuvre.**[1,20]

(i)   This has already been mentioned in connection with oesophageal or gastric varices and tears.

(ii) In any other patients in whom torrential bleeding persists and in whom surgery is not desirable or possible, one of two manoeuvres is helpful.

   (a) If the lesion is acute and superficial, or in the territory of mesenteric perfusion, bleeding may be controlled by vasopressin 0.2–0.4 i.u./min given for up to 36 h.
   (b) If the lesion is chronic, arterial embolisation via the catheter is probably the treatment of choice.
   (c) Stopping the bleeding by arteriography can sometimes be useful as a preliminary to surgery.

(5) **General measures.**

(i)   The patient should be allowed to take fluids as required and is offered a liberal soft nutritious diet with Maalox 20 ml every 2 h. Both these help neutralise stomach contents.

(ii) Sedation should be given to an anxious patient. Restlessness, which is often a manifestation of hypoxia, may respond to O_2 and transfusion. Remember the potential danger of O_2 therapy before giving it (see p. 71).

(iii) Measure the urinary output, as renal failure may occur in gastrointestinal bleeding.

REFERENCES

1   Allison D. J., Hemingway A. P., Cunningham D. A. (1982). Angiography in gastro-intestinal bleeding. *Lancet*; **ii:** 30.

2   Barer D. *et al.* (1983). Cimetidine and tranexamic acid in the treatment of acute upper G.I. bleeding. *N. Engl. J. Med.*; **308:** 1571.

3   Beckley D. E., Casebow M. P. (1986). Prediction of rebleeding from peptic ulcer; experience with an endoscopic doppler. *Gut*; **27:** 96.

4   Dick H., Porter J. (1978). Drug induced gastro-intestinal bleeding. *Lancet*; **ii:** 87.

5   Foster D. N., Miloszewksi K., Losowsky M. S. (1976). Diagnosis of Mallory–Weiss lesions. *Lancet*; **ii:** 483.

6   Freeman J. G., Cobden I., Lisham A. H. (1982). Controlled trial of glypressin versus vasopressin in the early treatment of oesophageal varices. *Lancet*; **ii:** 66.
7   Gillespie I. E. (1986). Bleeding oesophageal varices. *Br. Med. J.*; **292:** 1479.
8   Langman M. J. S. (1985). Upper G. I. bleeding: the trial of trials. *Gut*; **26:** 217.
9   Leader (1974). Erosive gastritis. *Br. Med. J.*; **3:** 211.
10   Leader (1982). Laser coagulation in bleeding peptic ulcers: passing gimmick or life-saving advance? *Lancet*; **ii:** 804.
11   Leader (1984). Bleeding oesophageal varices. *Lancet*; **i:** 139.
12   Leader (1984). Bleeding ulcers: scope for improvement? *Lancet*; **i:** 715.
13   Morris D. L. *et al.* (1984). Optimal timing of operation for bleeding peptic ulcer: prospective randomized trial. *Br. Med. J.*; **288:** 1277.
14   Pitcher L. J. (1971). Safety and effectiveness of the modified Sengstaken–Blakemore tube—a prospective study. *Gastroenterology*; **61:** 291.
15   Somerville K. W. *et al.* (1985). Somatostatin in the treatment of haematemesis and melaena. *Lancet*; **i:** 130.
16   Steer M. L., Silen W. (1983). Diagnostic procedures in G.I. haemorrhage. *N. Engl. J. Med.*; **309:** 646.
17   Storey W. D. *et al.* (1981). Endoscopic prediction of recurrent bleeding in peptic ulcers. *N. Engl. J. Med.*; **305:** 915.
18   Swain C. P. *et al.* (1986). Controlled trial of Nd-Yag laser photocoagulation in bleeding peptic ulcers. *Lancet*; **i:** 1113.
19   Triger D. R. (1986). Management of bleeding oesophageal varices. *Br. J. Hosp. Med.*; **35:** 96.
20   Young A. E. (1981). Therapeutic embolization. *Br. Med. J.*; **283:** 1144.

Lower gastrointestinal bleeding [2,3]

DIAGNOSIS

We define lower GI bleeding as bleeding occurring from a site below the ligament of Trietze. The usual presentation is the passage of fresh, bright red or maroon blood per rectum. However, malaena can occur from colonic bleeding (probably due to slow transit through a sluggish colon) and fresh blood per rectum can occur from torrential upper GI bleeding. It is therefore important to exclude upper GI bleeding in these patients. This is most easily done by passing a nasogastric tube. If you aspirate bilious, but blood-free fluid through this, you can be confident that there is no upper GI source. If there is no bile in your blood-free aspirate, you should undertake an upper GI endoscopy to ensure that the duodenum is not the site of haemorrhage.

The causes of lower GI bleeding are essentially colonic, the common ones being as follows.

(1) Diverticular disease. About 50% of the population aged over 60 years have diverticular disease, so to implicate it as a source of bleeding you really have to demonstrate a bleeding diverticulum. Bleeding usually occurs in a patient without previous symptoms from diverticular disease in the right colon. Treatment is surgical.

(2) Angiodysplasia. This vascular abnormality is an abnormal clustering of dilated submucosal veins and arteries. There is often thinning of the overlying mucosa, and the lesions are usually in the caecum and right side of the colon. They may be recognised on colonoscopy as prominent vessels, which, unlike normal colonic vessels, are wiggly rather than straight.

(3) Colorectal cancer.

(4) Ischaemic colitis.

(5) Colonic polyp.

(6) Inflammatory bowel disease (see p. 120).

(7) Small bowel lesions, between the ligament of Trietze and the ileum, are very uncommon causes of lower GI bleeding. The most frequent are tumours which may bleed, and in these patients there is usually a preceding history of abdominal pain and weight loss.

MANAGEMENT

(1) Initial resuscitation is as for upper GI bleeding (see p. 106).
(2) Thereafter, your aim is to arrive at a diagnosis of the site of the bleeding. Clinical indications are unfortunately not very helpful, and we recommend that the following investigative steps should be undertaken as a matter of urgency.

    (i)   Sigmoidoscopy. An estimated 10% of patients with lower GI bleeding have anorectal lesions visible on sigmoidoscopy.

    (ii)   If sigmoidoscopy is negative, colonoscopy is the next best investigative tool.[1] This should be undertaken urgently—the earlier the better. In a bleeding patient, oral preparation using 500 ml of 10% mannitol, 10 mg of metaclopramide, and plenty of water, should be commenced immediately. The bowel is usually clear enough to observe within 2–3 h.

    (iii) If the colonoscopy is negative, or the bleeding is too brisk to allow effective visualisation of the colon, two choices are open to you.

        (a) Technetium scintiscan. This technique is useful for localising the site of bleeding. A decision can then be made to operate, or direct further investigations.

        (b) Mesenteric angiography. This usually identifies the bleeding site only if the rate of loss is 0.5 ml/min, so is an ideal investigation in brisk bleeding.

(3) Having identified the site of the bleeding, the treatment is usually expectant or surgical. Colonoscopic electrocoagulation of bleeding sites and injection of vasopressin or gel-foam through an appropriately located intra-arterial catheter are further possibilities.

REFERENCES

1   Brandt L. J., Boley S. J. (1984). The role of colonoscopy in the diagnosis and management of lower intestinal bleeding. *Scand. J. Gastroenterol.*; **19** (Suppl. 102): 61.

2   Burakoff R. (1985). A case of haematochezia. *N. Engl. J. Med.*; **312**: 427.

3   Colacchio J. A. *et al.* (1982). Impact of modern diagnostic methods on management of active rectal bleeding—10 year experience. *Am. J. Surg.*; **143**: 607.

Acute pancreatitis [1,2]

DIAGNOSIS

(1) Acute pancreatitis causes pain, usually in the epigastrium or hypochondrium, associated with vomiting.

(2) A serum amylase of >1200 i.u./l (normal value 70–300 i.u./l) in this setting is diagnostic.

(3) Lipase, catalase and phospholipase levels are not additionally helpful. Trypsin, being specific to the pancreas, may become diagnostically more important.

(4) Acute pancreatitis may be associated with the following.

    (i)   Gallstones (50%). The likely cause is back pressure due to a stone blocking the common pancreaticobiliary duct.

    (ii)   Alcohol (10%). Here acute pancreatitis is superimposed on chronic pancreatic damage.

    (iii) Occasionally, hypercalcaemia, hyperlipidaemia and drugs may be associated with an acute attack.

    (iv) In 23% the cause is unknown.

(5) A raised amylase sufficient to cause diagnostic confusion can occur in small bowel obstruction, perforated duodenal ulcer, mesenteric infarction and dissection of the aorta. These can usually be distinguished clinically. Where genuine doubt exists, a laparotomy may have to be undertaken, but is associated with increased mortality and morbidity if the diagnosis turns out to be acute pancreatitis.

MANAGEMENT

(1) As the course, treatment and prognosis of mild and severe case differ, the first step is to determine the severity of the disease This is often difficult to assess clinically, but fortunately an objective assessment of severity is available.[3,5] The list below i of adverse prognostic factors in acute pancreatitis. If three o more of these are present within 48 h of your patient's admission, a severe attack is confirmed.

Adverse prognostic factors.

- (i)   WBC $>15 \times 10^9/l$.
- (ii)   Glucose >10 mmol/l (in a patient who is not a known diabetic).
- (iii) Urea >16 mmol/l (after correction of dehydration with i.v. fluids).
- (iv) $P_{aO_2} <60$ mmHg (8.0 kPa).
- (v)   Calcium <2.0 mmol/l.
- (vi)   Albumin <32 g/l.
- (vii) LDH >600 units/l.
- (viii) ALT >200 units/l.

More than three of these may be present within a few hours of admission, so you do not always have to wait 48 h to categorise your patient. Approximately 33% of patients are classified as 'severe'.

(2) A less frequently used method of assessing severity is to undertake a diagnostic peritoneal tap. If one or more of the following is present, you are dealing with severe pancreatitis.

- (i)   More than 20 ml ascitic fluid.
- (ii) Dark-coloured ascitic fluid.
- (iii) One litre of saline is infused and then withdrawn. If this lavage fluid is dark coloured, this is a good pointer to severity.

Having assessed the severity, any further treatment which is necessary can be based on a rational foundation.

SUPPORTIVE THERAPY

All patients with pancreatitis require basic supportive therapy, as outlined below. Further measures (8–10) should only be considered in the severe cases.

(1) Intravenous fluids. Patients with pancreatitis have a relative fluid deficiency and require i.v. saline replacement under CVP control. If this crystalloid infusion does not restore perfusion, colloid may also be required.

(2) Bowel rest. Although in mild cases there is no specific proof that strict bowel rest helps, we advocate a policy of nil by mouth, combined with nasogastric suction in all cases.

(3) Antibiotics. We reserve antibiotics for proven infection.

(4) Analgesics. Pancreatitis is an extremely painful condition. Adequate analgesic with pethidine 50–100 mg as required should be given.

(5) Oxygen therapy. A low PaO_2 is a feature of severe pancreatitis, and respiratory failure the commonest cause of death. The cause of the hypoxia is unknown. If humidified O_2 is not effective in restoring the PaO_2 to above 60 mmHg (8.0 kPa), IPPV should be instituted.

(6) Correction of renal insufficiency. If a poor renal output (<30 ml/h) persists in spite of adequate fluid replacement, you should try to promote a diuresis by using either mannitol, frusemide or dopamine (see p. 16). To ensure accurate measurement of urine output, you should catheterise the patient on admission.

(7) Correction of hypocalcaemia. This is probably secondary to the various peptides present, but is often associated with hypo-albuminaemia. It often corrects if you assiduously replace albumin (up to 40 g/day may be required) in the form of plasma, plasma protein derivatives or albumin; 10 ml of i.v. calcium gluconate may also be given.

Further measures

Most of the mild cases of pancreatitis respond to the supportive measures outlined above. In the severe case, additional therapeutic manoeuvres have been tried, but, as mentioned below, found to be unhelpful.

(8) Trasylol and i.v. glucagon. Controlled trials have not supported the use of these.

(9) Peritoneal lavage with hourly 2 l cycles of peritoneal dialysis fluid does not improve the outcome in patients with severe disease.

(10) Surgery. There is now little enthusiasm for total pancreatotomy or pancreatic debridement, which may however be necessary in an unresolving case as a delayed procedure. However, two studies have shown that if gallstones are involved in provoking pancreatitis, biliary surgery within 48 h of admission is very helpful.[4] You should therefore arrange ultrasound examination for gallstones early in the course of the illness.

REFERENCES

1 Bateson M. C. (1986). Acute pancreatitis. *Br. Med. J.*; **292:** 850.
2 Corfield A. P. *et al.* (1985). Acute pancreatitis: a lethal disease of increasing incidence. *Gut*; **26:** 724.
3 Corfield A. P. *et al.* (1985). Predictions of severity in acute pancreatitis: prospective comparison of three prognostic indices. *Lancet*; **ii:** 403.
4 Pellegrini C. (1985). The treatment of acute pancreatitis: a continuing challenge. *N. Engl. J. Med.*; **312:** 436.
5 Williamson R. C. N. (1984). Early assessment of severity in acute pancreatitis. *Gut*; **25:** 1331.

Ulcerative colitis[3,5,6]

Ulcerative colitis is characterised by widespread superficial ulceration of the colonic mucosa. It is a relapsing disease marked by episodes of bloody diarrhoea. The severity of any single episode is related to the extent of colon involved and, to a lesser degree, the severity of mucosal ulceration. In about 70% of episodes the colonic involvement is restricted to the sigmoid and rectum. Such cases do not usually constitute medical emergencies. However, more extensive involvement of the colon can give rise to a fulminant and potentially fatal disease. Appropriate management depends on accurate assessment of the severity of the attack.

DIAGNOSIS AND ASSESSMENT OF SEVERITY

(1) The diagnosis of ulcerative colitis is made by the association of the following.

    (i)   Clinical features (see below).

    (ii)   Sigmoidoscopic appearances. As the rectum is involved in 95% of all cases, sigmoidoscope evidence of the disease will almost always be present in an acute attack. The mucosa will be uniformly oedematous and red, there will be multiple small ulcers (often rather difficult to see macroscopically) or petechial haemorrhages, and free pus in the lumen of the bowel. The colonic mucosal wall will bleed on contact, and biopsy will provide histological evidence of the disease.

           Sigmoidoscopy must be carried out on all patients with a fresh attack of ulcerative colitis as it is the quickest and easiest way of substantiating the diagnosis.

   (iii) Barium enema abnormalities. In severe colitis, it is safe to perform a limited enema on an unprepared patient. Run in a small quantity of barium, remove it, and then insufflate a little air. This provides a good double contrast enema, and will help you diagnostically as well as giving an indication of the extent and severity of colonic involvement.

120

(2) The following features are helpful in identifying a severe attack.

   (i)   More than six liquid, bloodstained stools in 24 h. Patients with mild colitis frequently pass blood separately from faeces and it is the association of liquid faeces and blood which is important here.
   (ii) Fever. A mean evening temperature of greater than 38°C.
   (iii) Tachycardia. A mean pulse rate greater than 90 beats/min.
   (iv) Anaemia. This is usually a combination of the anaemia of chronic disease and the anaemia of blood loss. Hb levels below 10.0 g/100 ml indicate serious disease.
   (v)   ESR above 30 mm/h.
   (vi) Hypoalbuminaemia. Patients with ulcerative colitis may exude up to 30 g/day of protein through their raw colonic mucosa.
   (vii) Electrolyte disturbances. Electrolyte and fluid loss through the inflamed mucosa may also be considerable, and hypokalaemia, hypocalcaemia and hypomagnesaemia all occur.
   (viii) Abdominal pain. Pain prior to, and relieved by, defaecation is common in all grades of severity. Central abdominal pain and colonic tenderness on palpation usually indicate a severe attack.
   (ix) Straight x-ray of the abdomen. Dilatation of the colon (>6 cm), mucosal islands, and gas under the diaphragm in a patient with severe colitis are all indications for immediate surgery.
   (x)   It should be noted that the systemic complications of ulcerative colitis (arthropathy, skin rashes, iritis and liver disease) do not necessarily relate to the severity of the bowel involvement.

DIFFERENTIAL DIAGNOSIS

Bloody diarrhoea and systemic disturbance may be features of the following conditions.

(1) Amoebic dysentery. A history of foreign travel, characteristically foul-smelling stools, the typical undermined ulcer on sig-

moidoscopy and a positive amoebic complement fixation test will help you. Amoebae in the stools must be specifically looked for as they are easily confused with white cells.

(2) Dysentery. Usually caused by gram-negative bacteria of the *Shigella* or paratyphoid groups. Send stool and a rectal biopsy specimen for cultures and enquire after contacts. This disease may produce rectal changes indistinguishable from ulcerative colitis on sigmoidoscopic examination, as may campylobacter colitis.

(3) Crohn's disease. Classically, Crohn's involvement of the colon is patchy and the ulcers are deeper and serpigenous. However, as the management of acute Crohn's colitis is essentially the same as that of acute ulcerative colitis, the differentiation of these two conditions is not an immediate priority.

(4) Pseudomembranous colitis. In this form of colitis, which characteristically occurs in an ill patient who has been given antibiotics, particularly clindamycin, yellowish adherent plaques are seen on sigmoidoscopy. The likely causal agent is *Clostridium difficile*, and the illness responds well to metronidazole 400 mg t.d.s. or vancomycin 125 mg orally 6-hourly.[2] It is worth remembering that *Cl. difficile* may provoke a relapse of ulcerative colitis.[1]

The rectal bleeding in ulcerative colitis is not usually severe. This, plus the characteristic sigmoidoscope findings, serves to distinguish it from several other conditions which may present with severe rectal bleeding, such as ischaemic colitis, diverticular disease, carcinoma of the colon and haemorrhoids (see p. 115).

MANAGEMENT

(1) Like most GI emergencies, management is best undertaken jointly by physicians and surgeons.

(2) Take blood for FBP and ESR, serum Fe and folate, albumin and liver function tests, electrolytes including CA^{2+} and Mg^{2+} and urea. Do a daily, straight x-ray of the abdomen. Culture blood and stool.

(3) Correct the metabolic disturbances.

  (i)   The fluid disturbances. Anorexia, pyrexia and enteric losses give rise to considerable fluid electrolyte and protein depletion. Initial replacement should be with 0.9% N saline (154 mmol/l), preferably under CVP control. Hypoproteinaemia may be treated by colloid-containing fluids, for example 2 units of plasma or its equivalent, every 24 h.

(ii) Electrolytes.

    (a) Na^+ deficiency is corrected as above.

    (b) Plasma K^+ is usually low. If less than 3.5 mmol/l, give 3 g KCl (39 mmol) in each litre of replacement fluid. Otherwise remeasure 6 h later and replenish as indicated.

    (c) If the plasma Ca^{2+} is less than 2.3 mmol/l, give 10 ml 10% calcium gluconate solution (2.25 mmol/day).

    (d) If the plasma Mg^{2+} is below 1.0 mmol/l give 1 ml of 50% magnesium sulphate solution (2.0 mmol/day).

(iii) The anaemia. This is best corrected by blood transfusion. It is reasonable to aim at a haemoglobin level of 11.0 g/100 ml.

(iv) Nutrition. A recent controlled trial showed that there was no difference in patient outcome when either parenteral or oral nutrition was used. So only use parenteral nutrition if oral nutrition is not possible.[4]

(4) Suppressing the inflammation. If there is no indication for immediate surgery (see below), give:

(i) prednisone 60 mg i.v./day—this is the drug of choice;

(ii) antibiotics: the role of bacteria in either initiating or exacerbating ulcerative colitis is unclear. Bacteraemia in association with severe ulcerative colitis is common, and some authorities advocate the routine use of metronidazole, penicillin and gentamicin (see pp. 309–11).

    Salazopyrine does not confer additional benefit in an acute attack and causes anorexia.

(5) Surgery. In most severe cases of colitis a trial of medical management is preferable. However, if the patient is not improving by 10 days or at any stage deteriorates, total colectomy should be undertaken. The exact timing of such an operation has to be decided between physician and surgeon. However, immediate surgery is always required in the presence of the following conditions.

(i) Toxic dilatation of the colon. This diagnosis is suspected when prostration accompanies a distended and tympanitic abdomen and is confirmed by a straight x-ray of the abdomen. The widest diameter of the colon should be less than 6 cm. Toxic dilatation occurs only when virtually the entire epithelium of the colon has been destroyed. Mucosal islands or pieces of stripped off epithelium may hang from the colonic wall and be visible on the straight x-ray. This mucosal island sign is a further important pointer to immediate surgery.

(ii)   Perforation. Colonic perforation may not cause specific symptoms or signs but is associated with a general clinical deterioration. The diagnosis is confirmed by the presence of air under the diaphragm on an upright abdominal x-ray.

(iii) Profuse haemorrhage. This is, however, extremely uncommon, even in severe colitis.

(6) It is worth stressing again that treatment of this disease requires a combined medical and surgical approach. Initial treatment with prednisone neither precludes nor complicates later surgery.

REFERENCES

1   Dickinson R. J. *et al.* (1985). Double blind controlled trial of oral vancomycin as adjunctive treatment in acute exacerbations of idiopathic colitis. *Gut*; **26:** 1380.

2   Keighley M. R. B., Burrow D. W., Arabi Y. *et al.* (1978). Randomised control trial of vancomycin for pseudomembranous colitis and post operative diarrhoea. *Br. Med. J.*; **2:** 1667.

3   Lennard-Jones J. E. (1984). Medical treatment of ulcerative colitis. *Postgrad. Med. J.*; **60:** 797.

4   McIntyre P. B. *et al.* (1986). Controlled trial of bowel rest in the treatment of severe acute colitis. *Gut*; **27:** 481.

5   Truelove S. C., Jewell D. P. (1974). Intensive intra-venous regime for severe attacks of ulcerative colitis. *Lancet*; **i:** 1067.

6   Truelove S. C., Willoughby C. P., Lee E. C. G. *et al.* (1978) Further experience in the treatment of severe attacks of ulcerative colitis. *Lancet*; **ii:** 1086.

Medical conditions which may present with acute abdominal pain[2,4]

DIAGNOSIS

Abdominal pain may arise from stretching, violent contraction, ischaemia or infarction of the viscera, or from muscle, skin, bone, blood vessels, and nerves overlying or adjacent to the abdomen. It is not, therefore, surprising that many medical conditions can give rise to abdominal pain, and cause diagnostic confusion with an acute 'surgical' abdomen. In any patient presenting with abdominal pain, a careful history and a pause for reflection while necessary investigations are being performed and, where indicated, a trial of medical therapy is undertaken, may make an occasional laparotomy unnecessary. The following group of conditions should be considered.

(1) Intrathoracic causes. As the lower six thoracic nerves supply both thorax and abdominal wall, and as the heart and pericardium rest on the diaphragm, thoracic problems often cause abdominal pain—usually in the upper abdomen.

Important causes are:

(i) myocardial infarction (see p. 3).
(ii) pericarditis,
(iii) pulmonary embolus (see p. 47),
(iv) pleurisy,

all of which have characteristic clinical, radiographic, and ECG findings. A useful clinical tip here is that if unilateral abdominal pain arises from intrathoracic causes, palpation of the other side of the abdomen does not increase pain, whereas it will if the source is intra-abdominal.[2]

(2) Intra-abdominal and retroperitoneal causes.

(i) Acute pancreatitis (see p. 116).
(ii) Congestion of the liver, occurring in congestive cardiac failure and acute hepatitis, both of which should be looked for.
(iii) Acute pyelonephritis. This typically causes loin pain and frequency, but sometimes the pain may be confined to the bladder area. Examine a fresh midstream urine (MSU) under the microscope and send urine for culture.

(iv) Bowel ischaemia, which may be due to the following:

(a) Sickle cell disease. This should be considered in anyone of African or Mediterranean extraction with a history of jaundice. The patient may have parietal bossing and a characteristic facies.

(b) Henoch–Schönlein purpura. Abdominal pain may occur before the other signs, such as joint pains, rash, haematuria and rectal bleeding, appear.

(c) The vasculitic lesions of polyarteritis nodosa, systemic lupus erythematosus, and other allied conditions may give rise to bowel pain. Given the clinical setting, the diagnosis is usually obvious.

(d) The commonest cause is atheromatous narrowing of the mesenteric vessels.

(v) Constipation. This can, of itself, cause severe abdominal pain, especially in the elderly. Rectal examination and a straight x-ray of the abdomen will reveal all.

(vi) Infection.

(a) Gastroenteritis causes colic, usually in association with diarrhoea and vomiting. A careful history will help you here.[1]

(b) Worms. Tapeworms can cause quite severe abdominal pain. Ova and cysts should be looked for in the stools if a history of infestation is elicited.

(c) Primary peritonitis. This is an uncommon condition, usually occurring in patients with ascites. It is particularly liable to occur in children with the nephrotic syndrome. Aspiration of the abdominal fluid may reveal a cloudy aspirate from which diplococci may be grown.

(d) Typhoid.

(e) Mesenteric adenitis.

(3) Metabolic and endocrine causes.

(i) Diabetes. You will diagnose this by finding glucose and ketones in the urine and a raised blood glucose. Of course, appendicitis can precipitate diabetic coma. However, it is reasonable to see if treatment of the diabetes relieves the pain within 4 h or so before proceeding to laparotomy.

(ii)   Hypercalcaemia. There may be a history of constipation, polyuria, polydipsia, renal calculi and mood disturbance. Look for the typical deposits of calcium at the corneoscleral junction.

(iii) Porphyria (usually of the acute intermittent variety). The urine contains increased quantities of porphobilinogen which is oxidised to porphobilin—a brownish-coloured substance—when the urine is allowed to stand for half an hour. Abdominal tenderness is usually mild and rigidity absent.

(iv)   Addison's disease. This may also cause vomiting, hypotension and peripheral circulatory collapse (see p. 174). The patient may have the characteristic pigmentation, and the diagnosis is confirmed by measuring the plasma cortisol.

(v)   Heavy metal poisoning, classically lead—look for the blue line on the gums; blood and urine lead levels and urinary corporporphyrins I and III are increased. Antimony, cadmium, arsenic and mercury may also cause abdominal pain.

(4) Neurogenic causes.

(i)   Compression of nerve roots by either malignancy or local degenerative lesions. The pain is usually band-like and may give risc to scgmental hyperaesthesia over the abdomen and local pain over the vertebrae.

(ii)   Tabes dorsalis. Attacks of vomiting associated with severe epigastric pain and lasting for several days may occur in tabes dorsalis. The presence of irregular pupils reactive to accommodation but not to light (Argyll Robertson pupils) and absence of knee jerks aid the diagnosis.

(iii) Herpes zoster. Pain and paraesthesia precede the rash by a few days. It is usually unilateral and segmental and should not really cause confusion.

(5) Psychiatric cause: Munchausen's syndrome. These patients present with convincing symptoms and signs of various acute conditions, often involving the abdomen, which may be covered with scars. When the patient is apprised of your suspicions, the symptoms and signs disappear and the patient rapidly takes his own discharge, usually resisting offers of psychiatric help.

MANAGEMENT

Management involves excluding those conditions mentioned above. Obviously they will not all be relevant in every case of acute abdominal pain, but it is suggested that whenever possible the following investigations should be carried out.

(1) A plain supine x-ray of the abdomen. A recent prospective evaluation indicates that an erect film is of no additional diagnostic help.[3]
(2) Chest x-ray.
(3) Blood film.
(4) Examine the urine for sugar, blood and pus cells.
(5) Serum amylase.
(6) ECG.

PARALYTIC ILEUS

The following should be borne in mind.

(1) Drugs, e.g. ganglion-blocking agents (especially mecamylamine and pentolinium), anti-Parkinsonian drugs and anticholinergic drugs (e.g. atropine).
(2) Hypokalaemia.
(3) Severe gastroenteritis.
(4) Certain spinal events, e.g. spinal fusion, prolapsed intravertebral disc and spinal fractures.

ACUTE GASTRIC DILATATION

Diagnosis

(1) This condition may occur in hyperglycaemia, after childbirth, abdominal injury, application of a spinal cast and occasionally after abdominal surgery.
(2) The abdomen is distended and uncomfortable and a succussion splash can be readily elicited. Sufficient fluid may accumulate in the stomach to cause hypovolaemic shock.
(3) If reflux of the stomach contents occurs into the oesophagus the condition may be complicated by inhalation pneumonia.

Management

(1) Take blood for haemoglobin and PCV, electrolytes and urea.

(2) Pass a nasogastric tube and empty the stomach. Usually more than 1.5 litres can be aspirated.

(3) Set up a drip, preferably with CVP line, and replace the fluid lost into the bowel with alternating bottles of 5% dextrose and N saline (154 mmol/l). Add 26 mEq KCl to each litre of fluid given.

(4) Check the electrolytes 6 h later and adjust the ratio of saline to dextrose and the potassium supplements in the usual way.

(5) If reflux of abdominal contents into the lungs occurs, a large dose of steroids may minimise the ensuing inflammation. Give solumedrone 2 g i.v. daily for 2 days (see section on aspiration pneumonia, p. 96).

REFERENCES

1   Blacklow N. R., Cukor G. (1981). Viral gastroenteritis. *N. Engl. J. Med.*; **304:** 397.

2   Cope Z. (1968). *The Early Diagnosis of the Acute Abdomen*, 13th edn. London: Oxford University Press.

3   Field S. *et al.* (1985). The erect abdominal radiograph in the acute abdomen: should its routine use be abandoned? *Br. Med. J.*; **290:** 1934.

4   Havard C. (1972). Medical states simulating the acute abdomen. *Br. J. Hosp. Med.*; **7:** 443.

Acute liver failure[4,9]

DIAGNOSIS

(1) This condition should be considered in any confused (see p. 289) or unconscious (see p. 314) patient.

(2) It may be due to the following.

(i) Serious disease in a previously healthy patient, e.g. viral hepatitis, profound surgical shock with or without gram-negative septicaemia, Weil's disease, paracetamol overdose, repeated halothane exposure, or carbon tetrachloride or mushroom poisoning. In this situation there are no signs of chronic liver disease, but there is an acute onset of progressive and severe encephalopathy associated with jaundice. You should look for clinical evidence of these.

(a) Flapping tremor, demonstrated with the hands in dorsiflexion. More common, however, is generalised muscle twitching.

(b) Hepatic fetor.

(c) Constructional apraxia, restlessness, delusions or hallucinations.

(d) Jaundice (which may appear only after your patient has become confused and delirious).

The mortality in this group is very high, particularly if coma has occurred.

(ii) A relatively minor stress to a patient with biochemical and clinical evidence of chronic liver disease. This is the commonest situation and may be precipitated by:

(a) gastrointestinal haemorrhage (see p. 105);

(b) surgery;

(c) acute alcoholism;

(d) acute infection;

(e) potassium depletion and alkalosis (usually due to over-vigorous use of diuretics;

(f) drugs—morphine, paraldehyde, short- and medium-acting barbiturates, acetazolamide and ammonium chloride;

130

(g) paracentesis abdominis—ascitic fluid should be tapped in small quantities for diagnostic purposes, and only in large quantities for relief of symptoms;

(h) constipation.

(3) Do not forget that the patient with cirrhosis may also get hyponatraemia due to the sick cell syndrome (see p. 133). There may also be features associated with the cause of the cirrhosis. This is particularly relevant in alcoholic cirrhosis. Here, delirium tremens, thiamine deficiency producing Wernicke's encephalopathy, other B vitamin deficiencies and epileptic fits may all contribute to the disturbances in consciousness.

MANAGEMENT

Although the principles of management of acute and acute on chronic liver failure are similar, the objectives are somewhat different. In acute liver failure, supportive measures are used to buy time for the liver to recover. In acute on chronic failure, however, the underlying damage will not usually be amenable to any specific therapy. Thus, measures appropriate to the management of acute liver failure may not always be appropriate in acute on chronic failure. Obviously decisions as to which measures are appropriate will be taken in the context of each individual case.

In all patients with liver failure, take blood for full blood picture, electrolytes and urea, and liver function tests including prothrombin time and plasma ammonia. Take arterial blood for blood gas measurements. Save serum for *Leptospira* antibodies and Australia antigen, in case these become relevant later on. An EEG which shows progressive slowing of the α-waves with increasing coma is a useful objective method for assessing developments, although this is not often very practical.

Further management details are given below.

(1) General care of the confused (see p. 289) patient. Sedation should be avoided if at all possible (see (6) below), but if you think sedation is necessary, give phenobarbitone 10 mg i.m., diazepam 5 mg i.v. or chlormethiazole (see p. 293).[8] Drugs included in (2)(ii)(f) above must *never* be given.

(2) Treatment of the cause. Specific treatments are few, exceptions being chronic aggressive hepatitis (steroids) and Weil's disease (penicillin).

Steroids are sometimes given in fulminating viral hepatitis but they have not been shown to increase the survival rate.

(3) Stopping or treating the precipitating or contributory factors mentioned above.

(4) Minimising or correcting the multiple effects of liver cell failure.[1]

(i) Minimising the protein load. The rationale behind this is that the four groups of substances which appear in increased amounts in liver failure, and are the leading contenders for causing coma, are protein-related metabolites.[10]

(a) Ammonia. This arises largely through bacterial action on proteins in the gut, and is usually converted to urea by the liver. It causes coma in experimental animals, but not all patients dying of liver failure have a raised ammonia level.

(b) Amines. Several amines, notably octopamine and phenylethanolamine, are present in increased amounts. It is conceivable that they act as false neurotransmitters in the brain.

(c) Amino acids. Amino acid profiles are abnormal in liver disease. The amino acid precursors of octopamine and phenylethanolamine are present in increased amounts, which may account for the increased levels of these amines.

(d) Gamma amino butyric acid (GABA), the principal inhibitory neurotransmitter in the normal brain, is greatly increased in liver failure, and is the present leading contender as the inducer of the neuro-psychiatric problem in liver failure.[10]

Therefore, give the following.

(a) A low protein diet (20–30 g/day).

(b) About 6.4 mJ (1500 kcal) as carbohydrates. This may be given either orally (e.g. 3–4 bottles of Hycal, each of which contains 425 kcal) or i.v. via a central venous catheter (e.g. 1200 ml of 33% of dextrose). This glucose infusion will, it is hoped, prevent the development of hypoglycaemia, a common occurrence in hepatic failure (see iv).

(c) Neomycin 1 g 4-hourly by mouth and lactulose in a dose just sufficient to cause diarrhoea and lower the faecal pH to below 6 (approx. 30 ml t.i.d.) to sterilise the gut. Lactilol, a disaccharide analogue of lactulose which is well tolerated, is becoming more widely available.[6]

(d) 60–180 ml of 50% magnesium sulphate by mouth as a purge.

A controlled trial of branched chain amino acid infusion showed that while the amino acid profile was corrected no other benefit occurred. These amino acids may have a calorific value, but should not be used routinely.

(ii) Correcting fluid and electrolyte imbalance.

(a) Do not give more than 2 litres of fluid per day.

(b) The serum sodium is usually low (120–130 mEq/l). If the patient is heavier than normal or if there is ascites or oedema, this probably reflects dilution and redistribution rather than depletion. Giving sodium in this situation exacerbates fluid retention. The treatment is restriction of fluids to not more than 400 ml per day. Complaints of thirst from the patient can be alleviated by giving lemons to suck. However, with prolonged dietary sodium restriction and intensive diuretic therapy, a true sodium depletion state can occur (serum sodium usually less than 120 mEq/l). In this situation, saline infusion may cause dramatic clinical improvement, but should never be undertaken without getting expert advice. Dilutional hyponatraemia is by far the commoner of the two and, if there is doubt, saline should not be given. Terminally, sodium enters the cells, causing a further drop in serum sodium. Do not attempt to correct this with hypertonic saline. The outlook at this stage is almost hopeless. Hydrocortisone 200 mg 6-hourly and an infusion of glucose, potassium and insulin which helps to re-establish the sodium pump may be given (see p. 17).

(c) Potassium. Dangerous hypokalaemia can occur and potassium chloride supplements are given in the usual way.

(iii)   Correcting coagulation defects.[5] These may arise for either of two reasons.

  (a) Inadequate manufacture of clotting factors by the liver. This is only correctable by infusion of blood or blood products. Fresh frozen plasm (FFP) which contains all the clotting factors is the infusion of choice. If the platelet count is low, either a platelet infusion or an infusion of fresh blood may be required. Vitamin K 15 mg i.m. should also be given, although theoretically it should not be of great value, unless there has been fat-soluble vitamin malabsorption because of bile salt deficiency. If more than 4 units of ACD blood are necessary, give 10 ml 10% calcium gluconate/l of blood, as these patients are said to be particularly susceptible to citrate intoxication.

  (b) Intravascular coagulation associated with acute hepatic necrosis. This can be recognised by the combination of bleeding tendencies and bruising, thrombocytopenia, prolonged prothrombin, thrombin, and kaolin–cephalin times, a low fibrinogen titre and raised titre of degradation products (see p. 302). Intravenous heparin and fresh blood are the treatment of choice in this situation. This is clearly hazardous and should only be undertaken in conjunction with your haematological colleagues.

    Remember that every time you damage a blood vessel, bleeding is encouraged. Therefore, be sparing of your assaults on your patient.

(iv)   Correcting the blood glucose.

  (a) Hypoglycaemia may occur. If this is present, give 25 g of dextrose i.v.; ensure that your patient is having adequate carbohydrate calories (see p. 144) and check the blood sugar by Dextrostix 4-hourly.

  (b) Alternatively, hyperglycaemia may be present. This rarely needs treatment, unless ketosis develops. It is treated in the usual way with insulin (see p. 153).

(v)   Correcting the effects of widespread peripheral dilatation. This may cause hypotension and/or acute renal failure. Its mechanism is obscure, and treatment difficult. You should set up a CVP line and ensure that the CVP is within the normal range (see p. 342). Then infuse dopamine, beginning at a dose of between 2 and 5 μg/kg per min and increasing as necessary to a dose of 20 μg/kg per min. At this level of infusion it causes vasoconstriction to all arteries except those in the brain and kidney.

(vi) Combating sepsis. Amoxycillin in the usual doses, 250 mg i.v. 8-hourly, is safe, but if gentamicin is used, blood levels should be monitored (see p. 310). Remember, septicaemia is common in acute hepatic necrosis, whatever the cause.

(vii) Minimising the occurrence of gastrointestinal haemorrhage from acute erosions. Give cimetidine 200 mg 6-hourly i.v. in 5% dextrose, which will maintain the pH of the stomach contents above 6.

(viii) Supporting respiration. Many patients with acute hepatic failure develop shock lung (see p. 91). They may therefore require early ventilation to maintain an adequate $P\text{a}O_2$.

(ix) Controlling cerebral oedema. This complication is now the commonest cause of death in acute liver failure. The oedema is difficult to control; we find 100 ml of 20% mannitol, given by bolus and repeated hourly until a water diuresis is achieved, is the most successful therapy available. Steroids are not helpful.[3]

(x) Lowering the concentration of circulating substances usually removed by the liver, e.g. ammonia. The following methods have been used.

(a) Exchange transfusion of about 10 units of heparinised blood. At the end of the exchange the heparin should be reversed by giving protamine. Alternatively, plasma exchanges may be undertaken. This involves taking blood and separating plasma from the red blood cells. The latter are returned together with fresh frozen plasma. This is equally time consuming but does not tax the Blood Transfusion Service. Blood may be taken from the inferior vena cava and returned to a major vein. Alternatively, two lines of an arteriovenous Scribner shunt may be used, or access to a major artery and vein may be obtained by catheterisation, using the Seldinger technique.

(b) Haemoperfusion over an activated charcoal column.[2]

    (c) Haemodialysis.
    (d) Cross-circulation.
    (e) Extracorporeal liver perfusion.

Steps (b)–(e) can only be undertaken by a specialist unit, whose advice should be sought. The purpose of using these various support measures is to buy time until adequate liver recovery occurs. However, controlled trials have not shown any of these methods to be consistently superior to conservative therapy.

(5) Liver transplantation continues in a few centres and may in time be a feasible proposition for some of the 200–300 patients dying of acute liver disease in Britain each year.

(6) Sedation. Patients with acute liver failure may become disorientated and violent for many reasons and you should ensure that there is no reversible cause, such as hypoxia, before using any sedation. If sedation is essential, the benzodiazepam group of drugs is safest. Diazepam, 5 mg i.v. by slow i.v. infusion, usually secures peace for all. As it is metabolised by the liver, the dosage should be kept as low as possible, and repeated as infrequently as possible.[8]

REFERENCES

1   Fraser C. L., Arieff A. I. (1985). Hepatic encephalopathy. *N. Engl. J. Med.*; **313:** 865.

2   Gimson A. E. S. (1982). Earlier charcoal haemoperfusion in fulminant hepatic failure. *Lancet*; **ii:** 681.

3   Hanid M. A., Davies M., Mellon P. J. (1980). Clinical monitoring of intracranial pressure in fulminant hepatic failure. *Gut*; **21:** 866.

4   Hanid M. A. *et al.* (1978). Prognostic value of the oculovestibular reflex in fulminant hepatic failure. *Br. Med. J.*; **1:** 1029.

5   Kelly D. A., Tuddenham E. G. D. (1986). Haemostatic problems in liver disease. *Gut*; **27:** 339

6   Lanthier P. L., Morgan M. Y. (1985). Lactilol in the treatment of chronic hepatic encephalopathy: an open comparison with lactulose. *Gut*; **26;** 415.

7   Leader (1973). Safe prescribing in liver disease. *Br. Med. J.*; **2:** 193.

8   Leader (1977). Sedation in liver disease. *Br. Med. J.*; **1:** 124 f.

9   Leader (1980). Biochemical monitoring of encephalopathy in liver disease. *Lancet*; **ii:** 783.

10   Leader (1984). Hepatic encephalopathy today. *Lancet*; **i:** 489

Acute renal failure

Acute renal failure (ARF) [1,2,8]

Acute renal failure may be defined as a sudden rise in urea with or without accompanying oliguria (less than 400 ml/24 h in an adult). It is customary, and helpful, to consider ARF as one of the following.

(1) Pre-renal.
(2) Renal (established renal failure).
(3) Post-renal.

(1) *Pre-renal.* A physiological response of the kidney to poor perfusion, which may be caused by:

 (i) hypovolaemia (the commonest situation): this may either be absolute, due to fluid or blood loss, or relative, as occurs, for example, in septicaemia, major overdoses, liver failure and pancreatitis;
 (ii) cardiac failure.

 In the initial stages of pre-renal failure, the kidneys' concentrating power is normal, and the urine produced is highly concentrated (Table 2). It is essential to recognise this since restoring perfusion will avert established renal failure (see below).

(2) *Renal.* Renal damage per se is characterised by considerable deterioration in renal function and concentrating power. The urine produced, therefore, is dilute and serves to distinguish renal from pre-renal failure (see Table 2). Established renal failure may be due to any of the following.

 (i) Acute tubular necrosis (ATN). The pathogenic mechanism is unclear,[7] but the following causes are involved.

 (a) Persistent impairment of renal perfusion.

Table 2　Urine differences in pre-renal and established renal failure

	Pre-renal failure	Established renal failure
Urine/plasma osmolality ratio	>1.5 : 1	1.1 : 1
Urine/plasma urea ratio	> 10 : 1	<4 : 1
Sodium (mmol/l)	< 10	>20

(b) Drugs and chemicals, including mercuric chloride, carbon tetrachloride, aminoglycosides, radiocontrast mediums, low molecular weight dextran[5] and many others.

(c) Circulating pigments, including haemoglobin (haemolysis), myoglobin (rhabdomyolysis), and bilirubin.

(d) Frequently, several causes coexist.

(ii) Acute interstitial nephritis.[4] Causes include:

(a) drugs, such as non-steroidal anti-inflammatory drugs: rifampicin, phenindione, ampicillin and sulphonamides are among those implicated;

(b) infections, such as leptospirosis, Legionnaire's disease and the haemorrhagic renal syndrome.

(iii) Acute glomerulonephritis. Either primary, or secondary to a systemic disease, such as SLE, PAN or Henoch–Schönlein purpura.

(iv) Haemolytic uraemic syndrome (HUS), including thrombotic, thrombocytopenic purpura. Characterised by disseminated intravascular coagulation (DIC), which obliterates the renal capillaries, and microangiopathic haemolytic anaemia.

(v) Tubular obstruction, due to myeloma, insoluble drugs (sulphonamides), uric acid nephropathy and oxalate crystals.

(vi) Hypercalcaemia (see p. 182).

(vii) Acute on chronic failure. A trivial insult to a chronically diseased kidney may produce acute renal failure.

(viii) Occlusion of the renal arteries (elderly adults) or veins (infants).

(3) *Post-renal.* Obstruction to urine flow, with consequent reduction in renal function, may occur in the following sites.

(i) Ureter: calculi, retroperitoneal fibrosis, and tumours, most commonly of cervix or bladder. Bear in mind the possibility of obstruction to a single kidney.

(ii) Urethra: prostatic hypertrophy or urethral stricture. If the obstruction is relieved, prompt and rewarding return of renal function can be achieved.

DIAGNOSIS

The diagnosis of ARF, as defined, is biochemical. The signs and symptoms of uraemia, drowsiness, nausea and twitching are often overshadowed by the underlying cause.

(1) The history may give clues of long-standing renal disease, such as polyuria and nocturia, and there may be stigmata of chronic renal failure, such as hypertension, anaemia, pigmentation, pruritus, or renal bone disease with characteristic radiological changes of periosteal resorption of the distal phalanges. In such cases the kidneys when visualised, may either be large (polycystic or hydronephrotic) or small and shrunken. If there has been no previous renal disease, the kidneys are of normal size. In HUS there is an anaemia and thrombocytopenia, and fragmented cells are seen in the blood film. Clotting factors are often normal.

(2) The following biochemical changes are usually present.

   (i) *Raised urea.* ARF is usually accompanied by a catabolic state; the urea deriving from excessive protein breakdown can only accumulate—serum creatinine is also raised to a relatively lesser degree.

   (ii) *Raised potassium.* Potassium, released from cells by acidosis, catabolism and the sick cell syndrome (see p. 133), accumulates and may cause fatal cardiac dysrhythmias.

   (iii) *Low sodium.* This is usually caused by fluid overload (dilution) or the sick cell syndrome (redistribution) as opposed to true sodium depletion.

   (iv) *Low HCO_3.* Metabolic acidosis is due to inadequate secretion of non-volatile anions (e.g. SO_4 and PO_4), inadequate renal tubular generation of HCO_3, and inadequate formation of NH_3, by the distal tubules. H^+ ion formation may also be increased in this situation by poor tissue perfusion and tissue damage.

(3) Whatever the cause of ARF, septicaemia is highly likely, as is circulatory overload and oedema from inappropriate fluid intake. Features of these conditions are usually clinically obvious.

MANAGEMENT

This is aimed initially at diagnosing and correcting reversible or predisposing factors, i.e. poor renal perfusion or post-renal obstruction. If these measures do not restore renal function (i.e. established ARF is present), further treatment is as indicated below.

(1) The work load of the kidney is reduced by minimising tissue breakdown and hypoperfusion.
(2) The metabolic sequelae of kidney failure are dealt with until renal function is restored.
(3) A specific diagnosis of the cause of ARF is made and appropriate therapy is given. This is not usually relevant to immediate management, and will not be discussed further.

Management is continued as follows.

(1) Take blood for electrolytes, urea, FBP (including platelets) clotting factors, blood cultures, serum Ca^{2+} and blood glucose. Send urine, if necessary obtained by catheterisation, for Na^+ urea and osmolality (see Table 2). This only requires a few millilitres of urine, takes a short time to do, and must be insisted upon. Take a straight x-ray of the abdomen to evaluate renal size and visualise calculi.
(2) Weigh the patient if possible.
(3) Rule out a pre-renal cause.

    (i) Assess the patient for renal underperfusion. Heart failure is usually obvious and requires conventional treatment. Hypovolaemia causing general tissue underperfusion may also be evident clinically, i.e. cool peripheries, tachycardia, hypotension (particularly postural hypotension), plus disturbances of consciousness. If there has been substantial fluid loss, there may be reduced skin turgor, and eyeball tension will be low. A dry mouth and tongue are significant only in the absence of mouth breathing. The urine shows the characteristics of pre-renal failure. However, assessment of hypovolaemia can be extremely difficult, particularly if it is relative hypovolaemia, so if there is any doubt, the CVP must be measured (see p. 341). If this confirms hypovolaemia appropriate fluid (saline, blood or plasma) must be given rapidly until the CVP is in the upper range of normal (see

p. 343). Occasionally this manoeuvre restores urine flow even when the urine has shown the characteristics of established renal failure, but in this situation restoration of tissue perfusion must be carried out with the greatest attention to signs of impending fluid overload.

(ii) If correction of hypovolaemia or obstruction does not lead to brisk diuresis, renal damage has occurred, and established renal failure is present.

(iii) Remember that hypovolaemia may be due to a hypo-proteinaemic state, such as the nephrotic syndrome, in which case circulating volume may be restored with 1 litre of salt-free albumin.

(4) Rule out a post-renal cause.

(i) Catheterise the bladder to ensure that urethral obstruction is not present. If the bladder is empty, insert 200 ml of 0.02% aqueous solution of chlorhexidine, and withdraw the catheter.

(ii) Obstruction higher up may be difficult to exclude, but a high-dose nephrotomogram[3] (0.2 ml/kg body weight of 40% sodium diatrizoate) will usually demonstrate the presence of dilated pelvicalyceal system. Until recently, this was the usual method employed to exclude obstruction, but it is now being increasingly replaced by abdominal ultrasound examination.[6] You should use whichever is most readily available. Either method will also show the size and number of kidneys. This is helpful because:

(a) small, possibly scarred kidneys indicate chronic renal disease;

(b) it is a necessary prerequisite for renal biopsy which may be helpful diagnostically.

A high-dose intravenous urogram (IVU) constitutes a large osmotic load, and may precipitate acute cardiac failure. Thus, metabolic and circulatory disturbances must be corrected before a high-dose IVU is undertaken (see below). When obstruction is confirmed, the surgeons must be contacted without delay. Alternatively, it may be possible to relieve the obstruction in the x-ray department with percutaneous nephrostomies.

Management of established ARF

(1) The precipitating condition will need treatment on its own merits.

(2) (i) Mannitol 25%, 50 ml i.v. over 2 h, or frusemide 500 mg i.v. over 1.5 h may initiate a diuresis, and by promoting the polyuric phase of renal failure, curtail the duration of the illness.

(ii) Mannitol can precipitate acute cardiac failure in patients who are already overloaded; frusemide must never be given to patients who are still hypovolaemic, as it may reduce tissue perfusion still further.

(iii) Dopamine 2.5 μg/kg per min may also be used to induce a diuresis, and although no clinical trials of its efficacy have been undertaken, we think it a valuable asset.

(3) Fluid balance. Fluid intake should be 500 ml plus fluid lost the previous day (bearing in mind diarrhoea, vomiting and leaking fistulae). A weight loss of up to 0.5 kg/day indicates appropriate fluid replacement and is due to tissue loss. Gross fluid overload is an indication for dialysis.

(4) Nutrition. Starvation is the commonest cause for continuing catabolism in ARF and every attempt should be made to provide 12.6 MJ (3000 kcal) as carbohydrate or fat per day. This will reduce the urea load and promote healing. High-calorie fluids, such as Caloreen 16.7 kJ (4 kcal)/g or Hycal 1.0 MJ (244 kcal)/100 ml, given with due attention to the necessity for fluid restriction, are suitable sources.

In low potassium, high carbohydrate diets, 20 g of protein/day is allowable. Parentrovite forte 10 ml i.v. or equivalent should be given daily. If the patient is being dialysed, a 60 g protein, high-calorie diet can be given, and constitutes one of the advantages of dialysis. Intravenous fluids should only be given if oral feeding is impossible. A CVP line inserted with due regard to sterility helps, as the solutions you will infuse are highly irritant to small veins; 50% dextrose 4.2 MJ (1000 kcal)/500 ml and 10% Intralipid 2.1 MJ (550 kcal)/500 ml are the most concentrated calorie sources and contain no electrolytes. Intravenous feeding may induce acute carbohydrate intolerance (common anyway in ARF) and blood glucose levels should be checked regularly.

(5) Potassium. This is often high and may reach dangerous levels (more than 7 mmol) which require treatment.

(i) The best emergency therapy is 10 ml of 10% calcium chloride i.v. This decreases the excitability of membranes rather than actually reducing the serum K^+.

(ii) Intravenous infusion of 500 ml 20% dextrose containing 25 units insulin over 2 h will reduce serum K^+ temporarily.

(iii) If there is acidosis and the patient is not overloaded, 75–100 mmol $NaHCO_3$ i.v. over 2 h will reduce serum K^+.

(iv) Ion-exchange resins, either orally or rectally, can be used for the less urgent situation. Calcium zeocarb 225 (15 g t.i.d.) is perhaps the best.

(6) Sodium. As discussed above, low serum Na usually indicates Na dilution and redistribution and is not an indication for saline infusion. Unless there is gross loss of electrolytes, none should be given in the oliguric phase of ARF. In practice, small quantities (less than 30 mmol of Na^+ or K^+/day) are unavoidable if nourishing food is provided.

(7) Acidosis. It is rarely possible to correct the acidosis, aside from correcting tissue perfusion and oxygenation. Life-threatening acidosis (pH <7.1) is an indication for dialysis as $NaHCO_3$, the appropriate corrective fluid, will exacerbate fluid overload. The $NaHCO_3$ may, of course, be given as part of any replacement fluid necessary (see p. 302).

(8) Infections. Many patients with ARF are septicaemic—common organisms being *Pseudomonas pyocyanea, Bacterium proteus, Escherichia coli* and *Bacteroides*. Before the results of the blood cultures are available it is wise to start a broad spectrum, preferably bactericidal antibiotic regimen, e.g. ampicillin 500 mg 6-hourly, and cloxacillin 250 mg 6-hourly. If a change of antibiotics is indicated, they may be used as follows.

(i) The aminoglycosides. Gentamicin is the traditional choice, but because it probably has less nephrotoxicity, netilmycin is our present choice. Both require you to monitor blood levels. The initial dose of gentamicin is 1–1.5 mg/kg in a single dose; that of netilmycin is 2–3.5 mg/kg. Further doses are given according to blood levels (see p. 310). Remember that frusemide enhances the toxicity of gentamicin.

(ii) Cefotaxime 2–4 g 8-hourly i.v., or chloramphenicol 500 mg 6-hourly may be used safely, and without blood level monitoring. Cefoxitin may also be used.

(iii)   Azlocillin, 4 g/day in two divided doses may be used.
(iv)   Fungal infections may supervene and should be looked for in blood cultures. The likely organism is *Candida*, acquired endogenously, and oral amphotericin lozenges, 1 q.d.s., should be given prophylactically. (For the treatment of candidal septicaemia, see p. 311.)
(v)   If *Bacteroides* is found, metronidazole, chloramphenicol or clindamycin should be used (see p. 311).
(vi)   Do not give tetracyclines as they raise the blood urea.

(9) Drugs. Many are excreted unchanged by the kidney. Before giving any drug to a patient in renal failure, make sure you know the appropriate dose. Drug levels are often available now—avail yourself of them. Maxolon 10 mg (1 ml) is a safe antiemetic, and diazepam a suitable sedative. Paracetamol is probably the safest mild analgesic to use. Pethidine and morphine can be used in normal dosage as necessary.

Scrutinise the drug sheet daily, as a deterioration in either renal function or the patient's general state may be drug related.

(10) Bleeding. Because platelet function is impaired, and your patient often very ill, bleeding, especially from the GI tract, is common. This is effectively prevented by the use of an H_2-antagonist, such as ranitidine 150 mg daily, or regular antacids (see p. 109).

(11) Pulmonary oedema. This is due to a combination of fluid overload leading to a raised left ventricular end diastolic pressure (see p. 39) and leaky capillaries, as in the ARDS (see p. 91). As indicated below, dialysis will be required, but you should first institute treatment as outlined in the relevant sections.

(12) General. The patient with ARF has a physically and psychologically debilitating illness. You must try to keep up his morale (yours as well).

Keep him as mobile and active as possible. Always have a therapeutic reason for any invasive techniques, both for the patient's peace of mind and for reasons of infection. Remember that the quality of nursing care is a major determinant of the ultimate outcome, and will be improved if the nurses understand what is happening (as much as you do).

(13) Dialysis. Haemodialysis or peritoneal dialysis facilitates control of uraemia, allows a more liberal diet, and tides the patient over while the kidneys recover.

Indications for dialysis are seldom absolute, but the following are general guidelines.

(i)   Cardiac failure, or fluid overload, in an oliguric patient.
(ii)   Serum K^+ greater than 7 mmol/l.
(iii) Blood urea >35 mmol/l.
(iv) Blood pH <7.1.
(v)   To create room for i.v. feeding if this is deemed necessary.

A deteriorating trend in your patient may require you to commence dialysis before the above figures are reached. The theory and practice of peritoneal dialysis, which can be carried out successfully in any general medical ward, are well described in *Nephrology for Nurses*.[2]

REFERENCES

1   Black D. A. K., Jones N. F. (1979). *Renal Disease*, 4th edn. Oxford: Blackwell Scientific.
2   Cameron S. J., Russell A. M. E., Sale D. N. T. *et al.* (1977). *Nephrology for Nurses.* London: Heinemann Medical.
3   Cattell W. R., McIntosh C. S., Moseley I. F. *et al.* (1973). Excretion urography in acute renal failure. *Br. Med. J.*, **2:** 575.
4   Curtiss J. R. (1977). Drug induced renal disorders. *Br. Med. J.*; **2:** 242.
5   Feest T. G. (1976). Low molecular weight dextran—a continuing cause of A. R. F. *Br. Med. J.*; **2:** 1300.
6   Leader (1984). Diagnosing obstruction in renal failure. *Lancet*; **ii:** 848.
7   Levinsky M. J. (1977). Pathophysiology of acute renal failure. *N. Engl. J. Med.*; **296:** 1453.
8   Parsons V. (1974). Renal aspects of intensive care. *Br. J. Hosp. Med.*; **11:** 843.

Endocrine

Diabetic ketoacidosis and coma[1]

DIAGNOSIS

(1) Diabetic ketoacidosis usually presents with polyuria and drowsiness (pre-coma) which may in a surprisingly short time, but usually over a day or more, progress to coma.

    (i)   The patient usually shows signs of:

        (a) sodium and water depletion—dry slack skin, tachycardia and hypotension, particularly posturally induced;

        (b) acidosis—deep sighing respirations;

        (c) ketosis—fetor and vomiting.

    (ii)   The clinical picture is sometimes confused with salicylate poisoning, which also shows reducing agents on Benedict's test. However, ketones, unlike salicylates, are volatile and are removed by boiling the urine. In any case, the demonstration of a substantially raised blood glucose (>20 mmol/l) clinches the diagnosis.

    (iii)   A notable symptom of diabetic pre-coma is abdominal pain, particularly in children. This and the finding of shifting areas of tenderness may obscure the signs of acidosis, ketosis and dehydration which are also usually present.

    (iv)   The picture is utterly unlike that of hypoglycaemic coma. The only thing they have in common is that they may both occur in diabetes. If there is any doubt, *never give insulin*. Instead, give 50 g of glucose i.v. as a diagnostic test. This will do little harm to the patient in hyperglycaemic coma (although it may cause a sharp rise in serum K^+), whereas insulin can kill a hypoglycaemic patient or cause severe irreversible brain damage.

(2) It should be thought of in any patient drowsy or unconscious following:

    (i)   surgery or other trauma;

    (ii)   myocardial infarction;

    (iii)   cerebral infarction.

(3) It may be precipitated by an infection, which should always be looked for and treated as necessary.

(4) Rarely, it may be caused by acute pancreatitis.

MANAGEMENT

If possible, the patient should be managed in an intensive care unit.

(1) The aim of management is to correct:

    (i) fluid loss—the average loss is 90–120 ml/kg;

    (ii) electrolyte losses—especially potassium (average loss 3 mmol/kg) and sodium (average loss 7–10 mmol/kg);

    (iii) hyperglycaemia;

    (iv) acidosis.

(2) The fluid loss, causing hypovolaemia and the symptoms mentioned in (1)(i) on p. 151, should be corrected gradually (over the first 12 h).

Too rapid correction of hyperglycaemia causes gross osmotic swings, and too rapid correction of the acidosis causes pH differences between the CSF and blood, both of which are potentially hazardous. Therefore, take the following steps.

    (i) Put up a drip. As in all hypovolaemic states, a CVP line is preferable, as it allows replacement of adequate (and often large) volumes of fluid with safety.

    (ii) Take blood for electrolytes and urea, Hb and PCV and arterial pH. Check for ketonaemia by dipping a Ketostix in plasma. This separates off the non-ketotic forms of diabetic acidosis (see below).

    (iii) Give i.v. fluids as quickly as possible until the CVP is normal and the patient is well perfused (usually 3–4 litres are necessary within the first 4 h). Thereafter, slow down the infusion rate to supply normal maintenance requirements and then keep the patient well perfused

        Give the first 2 litres as 0.9% N saline (154 mmol/l) and thereafter change to alternate bottles of 0.9% saline (154 mmol/l) and 5% dextrose. Some advocate colloid infusion, rather than crystalloid infusion, in the initial resuscitation of diabetics.[2] The case for their use remains unproven; we keep to the conventional crystalloid

loid regimen, using colloids only if hypotension persists after initial fluid replacement. Potassium will also be required (see below).

(iv) There are two commonly used regimens for giving insulin.[3] The easiest is to give a continuous low dose infusion of soluble insulin.[5] Make up 24 units of soluble insulin in 20 ml of N saline (**not** dextrose, which is acidic and may inactivate the insulin) and infuse at a dose of 6 units (5 ml of your solution)/h.

A constant infusion pump is ideal, but a paediatric giving set is a useful alternative. This dose of insulin causes an average fall in sugar of 4–5 mmol/l per h. The rate of fall will be slower in the presence of infection.

A less useful regimen is to give 6 units of soluble insulin i.m. each hour, following a loading dose of 20 units i.m.

It is unusual for patients to require more than 6 units of insulin/h. If they do, think of:

(a) infection;
(b) other endocrine problems, such as thyrotoxicosis or Cushing's syndrome;
(c) drug interaction: this is a particular problem in diabetic labour when very high doses (30 units i.v./h) may be required to maintain normoglycaemia if high doses of steroids or β-adrenergic agonists are being given.[6]

(3) While this is going on pass a urinary catheter. You will need this to ensure that an adequate urine flow is established (acute renal failure is very rare in diabetes, possibly because the osmotic diuretic effect of glycosuria 'protects' the kidney). Do not rely on urine glucose to monitor progress—frequent blood glucose measurements are essential for this purpose. Remember to remove the catheter as soon as the patient is better (which, it is hoped, should be within 24 h), taking a catheter specimen of urine for culture as you do so.

(4) Next, consider the following.

(i) Electrolyte losses. The polyuria preceding coma will have resulted in sodium and potassium depletion. Although the initial sodium is usually normal, the previous urinary losses have been hypotonic with respect to plasma. Hence, 5% dextrose may be given early in treatment (see

(2)(iii) above). The initial plasma potassium may be high because of intracellular acidosis, but will fall rapidly as the blood glucose falls and as the acidosis is corrected. Thus, even if the initial potassium is high, you are highly unlikely to run into problems with hyperkalaemia. The reverse is usually the case. One gram KCl (13 mmol K^+) may be given with the first litre of fluid and the first dose of insulin provided the T waves on the ECG are not peaked, and that urinary output is adequate; 2 g KCl (26 mmol K^+), given with each ensuing litre of fluid, is usually sufficient. Occasionally even more may be required, as shown by serial plasma K^+ estimations. The K^+ should be kept at around 4.5 mEq/l.

(ii) Acidosis. Although acidosis is itself dangerous, the routine administration of HCO_3 to patients with a pH of more than 7.1 is not recommended because of the risk of:

(a) paradoxical increase in CSF acidosis alluded to above;
(b) further increasing K^+ flux into cells.
When the pH is less than 7.1 give 50 mmol of HCO_3 in the first 2 h followed by 50 mmol in the next 4 h.
Remember to give extra K^+; we suggest 26 mEq K^+ for each 50 mmol of HCO_3.

(iii) The precipitating cause. Do an ECG, and if possible have a continuous ECG display to detect any arrhythmias or evidence of hyper- or hypokalaemia.
Look for infection, especially in the chest (chest x-ray) and urinary tract (urine microscopy and culture). Take blood cultures routinely and start the patient on a broad-spectrum antibiotic, such as ampicillin 500 mg q.d.s.

(iv) If your patient is comatose, aspirate the stomach content through a nasogastric tube, as many patients in diabetic coma have dilated, atonic stomachs, the contents of which may cause inhalation pneumonia. If there is no gag reflex you should protect the lungs with a cuffed endotracheal tube prior to aspirating the stomach.

(v) Continuing hypotension is almost certainly due to hypovolaemia. If it persists despite adequate fluid replacement, consider other causes of hypotension (see p 295) and treat accordingly.

(vi) General nursing care of the comatose patient (see p. 323).

(5) If you use the insulin regimen suggested above, the blood glucose is likely to be halved within 4 h—4-hourly estimates of blood glucose, electrolytes and arterial pH are therefore adequate.

(6) As a result of these and your other clinical measurements, you may have to adjust the following.

   (i) Sodium—by altering the ratio of 5% dextrose to N saline.
   (ii) Potassium—if the serum K^+ is normal, continue with the same dosage; if low, increase the dosage, and if high, stop the K^+ immediately but repeat the measurement as a high K^+ at this stage is extremely uncommon.
   (iii) Bicarbonate—if the pH is rising gradually, further administration of HCO_3 is unnecessary. If the pH is still dangerously low (i.e. less than 7.1) and not rising, you may have to give more HCO_3. Give this slowly (i.e. 75 mmol in the next 4 h).
   (iv) Fluid—you have probably not given the total replacement within 4 h, but remember to watch the patient's neck veins and lung bases as well as the CVP to ensure you do not give too much.
   (v) Phosphate—hypophosphataemia of a significant degree (PO_4 <0.32 mmol/l) occasionally occurs in diabetic ketoacidosis. It causes general debility and anergy, and may be corrected by infusing 9 mmol of monobasic potassium phosphate in 0.5% saline over 12 h, and repeating as necessary.[4]

(7) Four hours later, repeat the measurements. By now the patient should be considerably improved, and probably out of coma.
   If he is not, it may be for the following reasons.

   (i) It may just be that the patient's initial metabolic disturbances were very severe, and are not yet corrected;
   (ii) There may be an undetected precipitating cause of coma. Estimate the serum amylase and calcium at this stage, or before if there is a suggestive history of pancreatitis.
   (iii) He may have one of the following complications of the condition or its treatment.

      (a) Hypoglycaemia. Check that the blood glucose is not below 4.5 mmol/l (80 mg%).

      (b) Cerebral oedema.[7] Subclinical brain swelling, as seen
          on a CT scan, often occurs during the treatment of
          diabetic coma; overt cerebral oedema can occur. Its
          aetiology is uncertain, but it may be related to: too
          rapid lowering of blood glucose, or replacement of
          fluid loss with hypotonic solutions. This allows a high
          osmotic gradient to develop between extra- and
          intracellular compartments.
      (c) Hypokalaemia and/or gastric dilatation.
      (d) Major artery thrombosis.
      (e) Addison's disease. Diabetic ketosis may precipitate
          an Addisonian crisis in a patient with pre-existing
          adrenal insufficiency. Check the arterial pressure.

(8) Improvement in blood sugar levels often precedes improvement in other metabolic variables. Thus, the patient may be
normoglycaemic but still nauseated or vomiting and ketotic.
For this reason it is suggested that the insulin infusion rate
should be reduced to 3 units/h, and that 5% dextrose (1 litre
over 8 h) is given, as soon as the blood glucose is less than
11 mmol/l. This regimen is continued until the patient can eat
and drink normally. He should then start maintenance subcutaneous insulin. Assessing control by urine testing no longer
has a place in the management of acute diabetic emergencies,
and regimens of the sort outlined above are probably the
easiest way of controlling any diabetic who cannot eat and
drink, e.g. those undergoing surgery or labour (see p. 162).

(9) Remember that the gross desalination of hyperglycaemia can
mask signs of infection. These may become apparent when
your patient's fluid deficiencies have been corrected, so always
re-examine the patient carefully at this stage. Diabetic
ketoacidosis per se can cause a brisk leucocytosis, so is not in
itself a reliable sign of infection.

REFERENCES

General reading
Belchetz P. E. (1984). Endocrine emergencies. In *Clinical
Endocrinology*. (Keynes W., Fowler P. B., eds.). London
Heinemann Medical.

Specific

1   Foster D. W., McGarry D. J. (1983). The metabolic derangements and treatments of diabetic ketoacidosis. *N. Engl. J. Med.*; **309:** 159.

2   Hillman K. M. (1982). Crystalloid infusion in diabetes. *Lancet*; **ii:** 548.

3   Leader (1977). Insulin regimens for diabetic ketoacidosis. *Br. Med. J.*; **1:** 405.

4   Leader (1981). Treatment of severe hypophosphataemia. *Lancet*; **ii:** 734.

5   Page M. McB. *et al.* (1974). Treatment of diabetic coma with continuous low dose infusion of insulin. *Br. Med. J.*; **2:** 687.

6   Thomas D. J. B. *et al.* (1977). Salbutamol induced diabetic ketoacidosis. *Br. Med. J.*; **2:** 438.

7   Winegrad A. I. *et al.* (1985). Cerebral edema in diabetic ketoacidosis. *N. Engl. J. Med.*; **312:** 1184.

Hyperosmolar non-ketotic diabetic coma[1,2]

DIAGNOSIS

(1) Diabetic coma may occur without ketonuria in the following circumstances.

    (i)   When diabetic coma is complicated by acute renal failure. Here the patient has ketonaemia and is acidotic.

    (ii)   In diabetic coma with lactic acidosis (see p. 69).

    (iii)   In hyperosmolar non-ketotic diabetic coma. This is really rather a bad term, because diabetic ketoacidosis is also hyperosmolar—not, however, to the same degree. These patients have no ketones in the urine or blood, are not acidotic and do not, therefore, overbreathe.

(2) In (1)(iii) above, the patients frequently are elderly and have an insidious onset of illness over weeks. The illness may be provoked by thiazide diuretics or anticonvulsants. It may present with either focal or diffuse neurological signs, with or without an accompanying cerebrovascular accident. The blood glucose level is often very high (around 60 mmol), causing an osmotic diuresis in which large amounts of potassium, sodium and water are lost. The ensuing hypovolaemia is usually obvious clinically and is associated with pre-renal uraemia. There is proportionately greater loss of water than salt, and the serum sodium is often raised—above 155 mmol. The combination of a raised sodium, urea and glucose causes very high serum osmolality, which may exceed 400 mosmol/kg (serum osmolality (mmol/kg) = 2 [Na + K] + urea + glucose—all in mmol/l). This in turn causes severe intracellular dehydration—one of the factors responsible for coma. There is a good correlation between osmolality and the conscious state, as indicated below.

Plasma osmolality (mmol/l)	Conscious state
310–330	Alert
330–350	Obtunded
350–370	Stuporous
370–420	Comatose

(3) The pathogenesis of this illness is not fully established, but recent evidence suggests that these patients may have just sufficient circulating insulin to control lipolysis, thereby preventing the development of ketones, but not enough to prevent hyperglycaemia.[2] The prior use of thiazide diuretics which have an additional hyperglycaemic effect is common.

(4) Fifty per cent of these patients will have an obvious, and often serious, precipitating illness, such as infection, stroke, myocardial infarction or recent surgery.

MANAGEMENT

Take blood for haemoglobin and PCV, electrolytes and urea, blood glucose, serum amylase and calcium and plasma osmolality.

(1) Correct the following conditions as described.

(i)   Dehydration, hyperosmolality and sodium and potassium depletion. As mentioned in (2) above, the fluid and electrolyte loss in hyperosmolar coma is usually greater than that in ketotic coma. Loss of 25% of the total body water is common. You should aim to replace half this loss in the first 12 h, and the rest in the ensuing 24 h. The problem is with what. As so often, there is controversy. Some experts advocate using the same fluid and electrolyte regimen as in ketotic diabetic coma (see p. 152). However, the conventional advice is to replace the water and sodium deficit with 0.5 N saline from the onset. A sensible compromise is to use 0.5 N saline if the initial serum sodium is above 150 mmol/l, or if the sodium rises above 150 mmol/l at any stage during treatment, but otherwise to give isotonic saline as for ketotic coma. Remember, when calculating fluid deficits, that in old people the total body water is only 50%, not the more usual 60% of body weight.

(ii) Hyperglycaemia. It might be thought that the lack of acidosis allows full sensitivity to insulin. This is often, but by no means always, the case. Insulin should be given as described for ketotic diabetic coma, the response being checked with repeated measurements of the blood glucose, and the rate of administration adjusted accordingly.

(2) Venous and arterial thromboses are very likely to occur in this

situation, so heparinise the patient for 2–3 days (10 000 units i.v. 6-hourly—see p. 17).

(3) Treat any underlying or precipitating causes, such as infection or acute pancreatitis.

(4) After the acute episode has passed, these patients often have mild diabetes which can be controlled with diet alone or with small doses of oral hypoglycaemic agents.

REFERENCES

1   Arieff A. I., Carroll H. J. (1972). Nonketotic hyperglycaemic coma. *Medicine*; **51:** 73.

2   Gill G. V., Alberti K. G. M. (1985). Hyperosmolar non-ketotic coma. *Practical Diabetes*; **2:** 30.

Non-ketotic diabetic acidosis

The acidosis of diabetic pre-coma and coma is not always caused exclusively by ketones. It may occasionally be due to other anions: formic acid in mcthyl alcohol poisoning; a-ketoglutaric acid in liver failure; phosphate and other anions in renal failure; and lactic acid, which is much the most common. For this reason it is important to check that ketones are actually present in the plasma of a diabetic in acidosis. If they are absent, then these other serious underlying conditions should be looked for.

Urgent surgery in diabetics

There is an increased mortality in surgery undertaken in poorly controlled diabetics. Every diabetic has a 50% chance of undergoing surgery in his or her lifetime. As 5% of these are emergency operations, this is a problem which you may well be asked to attend to.

In any diabetic you should take the following steps.

(1) Discontinue the prevailing mode of therapy.
(2) Give 1 litre of 10% dextrose 12-hourly with 26 mmol K^+ added (see 6 below).
(3) Infuse insulin at a dose of 3 units/h with an infusion pump (see p. 153 and (5) below).
(4) Monitor blood sugar and adjust your insulin infusion accordingly (Table 3). You should do a preoperative sugar, intraoperative sugars at hourly intervals, and 3–4-hourly postoperative sugars.

Table 3

Sugar level (mmol/l)	Insulin infusion (units/h)
5	1
5–10	3
>10–20	4
>20	5

(5) Continue the regimen until the patient is eating again, and then switch back to the previous regimen (provided, of course, this was controlling the diabetes adequately!).
(6) You should also monitor the K^+ level.

(i) If the K^+ level is >5 mmol/l, stop the K^+ infusion.
(ii) If the K^+ is between 3.5 mmol/l and 5 mmol/l, add 26 mmol K^+ to each litre of 10% dextrose.
(iii) If the K^+ <3.5 mmol/l, add 52 mmol K^+ to each litre of 10% dextrose.

(7) There are some circumstances where you will need higher levels of insulin infusion.

(i)   If your patient has a severe infection.
(ii) In cardiac surgery (the bypass pump may be primed with dextrose).
(iii) If an adrenergic agent is being used at the same time.
(iv) If your patient is having parenteral nutrition.
(v)   If your patient is on suppressive doses of corticosteroids.

(8) Remember that if your patient is in diabetic ketoacidotic pre-coma, initial control of the metabolic state may:

   (i) relieve the abdominal pain and vomiting which you thought was surgical in origin;
   (ii) make any necessary surgery much safer.

   So always allow a few hours for correction of this (see p. 155) before undertaking surgery.

For elective surgery a somewhat different approach is permissible.

(1) Insulin-dependent diabetics.

   (i)   Admit 3 days prior to surgery.
   (ii) If they are not already on a twice-daily regimen of a mixture of medium- and short-acting insulin, change them to this.
   (iii) On the preoperative day, give only the evening soluble insulin.
   (iv) On the operative day, proceed as for emergency surgery with i.v. insulin and glucose.

(2) Non-insulin-dependent diabetics (NIDDs).

● Diet controlled
   (i) If fasting sugar is <7.0 mmol/l, you will not need to take any special action.
   (ii) But if major, and therefore prolonged, surgery is anticipated, or if the fasting sugar is >11.0 mmol/l, proceed as for emergency surgery with i.v. insulin and glucose.

● Tablet controlled
   (i) Stop the tablets the day before surgery, 3 days before in the case of long-acting sulphonylurea such as chlorpropamide.
   (ii) Assess control on day of admission, and then proceed as for 'diet controlled' above.

Hypopituitary coma[1]

DIAGNOSIS

(1) This may be precipitated in a patient with long-standing pituitary failure by infection, trauma (including surgery), myocardial infarction or cold, sedatives and hypnotics. It may also occur following an acute insult to the pituitary gland, e.g. surgery, head injury, haemorrhage or postpartum infection.

(2) The clinical picture is one of gonadotrophin, thyroid and adrenal deficiency.

These deficiencies have usually developed gradually, as have the patient's symptoms. Thus, there is a history of somnolence, sensitivity to cold and increasing confusion, progressing over a few weeks to coma. On examination, the skin is strikingly pale and dry, but of fine texture. Pubic and axillary hair are usually absent and the prematurely wrinkled features of hypogonadism may be obvious. The breasts and genitalia are atrophic. There is a general lack of pigmentation, and blood pressure, temperature and pulse rate are often below normal. If, in addition, the posterior pituitary is involved, polyuria due to lack of ADH may cause dehydration.

These multiple endocrine deficiencies all contribute to the coma, as indicated below.

MANAGEMENT

Estimate the blood glucose with BM stix and take blood for full blood count, electrolytes and urea, blood glucose, serum thyroxine, blood cortisol, growth hormone and arterial blood gases.

(1) Consider treatment of the possible causes of coma, of which the following are the most common.

    (i)   Hypothyroidism. Attempts to raise the metabolic rate with tri-iodothyronine (T3) while other causes of coma are still operative exacerbates coma, and this should not be given until treatment of other causes of coma is under way. A suitable regimen for the administration of T3 is:

0.02 mg 8-hourly for three doses; then 0.05 mg 8-hourly for three doses; then 0.1 mg 8-hourly thereafter. The drug is most usually given via a nasogastric tube, but can be given i.v. if the appropriate preparation is available.

(ii)   Hypothermia (see p. 265).
(iii) Electrolyte disturbances. Two patterns of electrolyte disturbance may occur.

   (a) Water intoxication. This is by far the most common and arises because, in the absence of cortisol, the patient's capacity to mount a water diuresis is depressed. If the posterior pituitary is intact, the inappropriate secretion of ADH associated with myxoedema may also be a factor. Water-intoxicated patients may complain of weakness, headache, nausea and blurring of vision. Tendon reflexes are exaggerated and muscle cramps occur. Drowsiness progresses to confusion, convulsions and coma. The serum sodium is usually less than 120 mmol/l, there may be hypokalaemia, and the urea is usually low (below 6.0 mmol/l). Intake of all fluids should be stopped, unless there is oliguria. This is frequently all that is necessary. However, if oliguria is present, if the patient is in pre-coma, or convulsions have occurred, give 2 N saline at about 40 ml/h until the urine flow has been more than 45 ml/h for at least 3 h.

   Because of the risk of water intoxication, you should not give hypotonic fluids to patients in hypopituitary coma until adequate replacement of cortisol and thyroxine has been achieved.

   (b) Salt and water depletion. This is uncommon. The serum Na^+ may be low, but the urea will be high and the patient hypovolaemic. When it is due to polyuria secondary to ADH deficiency, give 5 units of aqueous pitressin subcutaneously and sufficient N saline to make good previous salt losses. However, it is more commonly due to vomiting and diarrhoea occurring in a patient with cortisol deficiency. N saline infusions will again be required.

(iv) A CVP line will help considerably in the management of these electrolyte disturbances and you should insert one whenever possible.

(v) Hypoglycaemia. Give 25 g of dextrose i.v. (see p. 172). The problems in (iii) and (v) are primarily caused by adrenocortical insufficiency and at least 100 mg of hydrocortisone must be injected i.v. without delay (see p. 175). This may initiate a diuresis if water intoxication has occurred, or protect the patient from water intoxication if saline and water depletion require large volumes of intravenous fluid.

In addition the following may be contributory.

(vi) Hypoxia. Give 50–60% O_2 by face mask. If this is inadequate, as judged by the P_{aO_2}, intermittent positive pressure respiration is indicated.

(vii) Hypotension. This is usually due to steroid insufficiency and/or hypovolaemia and responds to hydrocortisone and adequate fluid replacement.

(2) Investigations and treatment of the cause.

(3) When coma has been relieved and the crisis is passed, daily replacement therapy will be necessary.[1]

(4) Diabetics who have been hypophysectomised for treatment of diabetic retinopathy are extremely sensitive to insulin—changes of a few units either way may lead to severe hypoglycaemia or ketoacidosis.

REFERENCE

1 Garrod O. (1967). Hypopituitary coma. *Hosp. Med.*; **2:** 300.

Pituitary apoplexy[1]

Pituitary apoplexy occurs when sudden haemorrhage and/or necrosis cause sudden expansion of a pituitary tumour.

DIAGNOSIS

(1) It presents with a characteristic array of symptoms and signs. There is a sudden onset of headache, bilateral amblyopia and ophthalmoplegia. The patient becomes stuporous and may lapse into coma. Neck stiffness may be present.
(2) A lumbar puncture should not be performed as this presentation is also consistent with temporal lobe herniation.
(3) Skull x-ray nearly always shows enlargement of the sella.
(4) CT scan of the head may show parasellar haemorrhage and suprasellar mass effect.

MANAGEMENT

Since the patient may die within hours, neurosurgical help should be sought urgently. The relief of pressure by a transnasal decompression of the sella is the procedure of choice. In the interval, give dexamethasone 6 mg i.v. every 6 h together with the usual measures as necessary to support circulation and ventilation.

REFERENCE

1   Riskind P. N. (1986). A case of pituitary apoplexy. *N. Engl. J. Med.*; **314:** 229.

Acute lactic acidosis[1,4,5]

Lactic acid, which is formed from pyruvate as the end-product of anaerobic glycolysis, is in equilibrium with pyruvate. The position of equilibrium is determined mainly by the tissue PO_2.

The lactate level, normally less than 1 mmol/l, will rise in the following circumstances.

(1) With a rise in the pyruvate concentration. Here the pyruvate lactate ratio is normal (1 : 10) and the patient is not acidotic. For reasons that are not understood, this occurs in the setting of hyperventilation such as may occur after a stroke or pulmonary embolus. The prognosis for these patients is that of their underlying disease, which should be treated in the normal fashion.

(2) With poor tissue oxygenation. Here lactate has risen ten times or more relative to pyruvate (the absolute level of lactate is >5 mmol/l) and the patient is acidotic. There are two separate categories.

    (i)   The decreased tissue oxygenation may be evident. The patient is seriously ill. The oxygen supply to the tissue is severely compromised, as in septic, cardiac or hypovolaemic shock, or hypoxia for any reason. In this group the excess blood lactate falls with therapy directed at reversing the underlying 'shock' state. (This group is the type A lactic acidosis of Cohen and Wood.)

    (ii)   Lactate production may be increased, or lactate removal decreased without any obvious oxygen supply problems. Thus, the patient initially appears to be well perfused with a normal Pao_2. The reason for this form of lactate disturbance, despite an apparently adequate oxygen supply, is not clear. In this group of patients (type B lactic acidosis of Cohen and Wood), there may be no obvious antecedent illness, but more commonly there is an identifiable provocative factor. The most important of these are that the patient may have been taking phenformin, suffer from ethanol intoxication, have had a rapid sorbitol or fructose infusion, or have severe liver disease. Occasionally the acidosis develops in patients who seem to be recovering satisfactorily from an event such as

168

myocardial infarct, and an increase in lactate may occur during the first few hours of treatment of diabetic ketoacidosis.

In this group, the serum lactate levels are uninfluenced by oxygen therapy, and the serum HCO_3 often fluctuates wildly, and with apparently only little relation to HCO_3 infusion. The decreasing use of phenformin has resulted in a decline in incidence of type B lactic acidosis as metformin is only very rarely associated with lactic acidosis.

DIAGNOSIS

(1) Lactic acidosis should be suspected in acidotic (and therefore hyperventilating) patients if a large number of anions remains unaccounted for (the anion gap).[3] The sum of the anions that we conventionally measure [Cl^- and HCO_3^-] normally approximates to the sum of the serum cations [Na^+ and K^+]. Thus, if the anion gap [$Na^+ + K^+$] − [$Cl^- + HCO_3^-$] is greater than 18 mmol/l, and is not accounted for by ketones, salicylates, uraemia, methanol, ethylene glycol or paraldehyde, all of which can give rise to a metabolic acidosis with a large anion gap,[2] lactic acidosis may well be present.

(2) The presence of lactic acidosis should, of course, be suspected in a diabetic patient who is acidotic but who has no, or only few, circulating ketones.

(3) It has been found that the PO_4 level is usually high in lactic acidosis. An average level of 2.9 mmol/l has been recorded, whereas in the metabolic acidosis of diabetic coma, the average is 1.6 mmol/l.

(4) If you can measure it, a lactate level of >5 mmol is arbitrarily considered as diagnostic. The average level in 285 cases of type B acidosis was 16.9 mmol/l, with an average anion gap of 37 mEq/l.

MANAGEMENT

Type A lactic acidosis

The excess lactate here is only one of degree, as most 'shock states' are accompanied by increased lactate levels. The treatment is that of the 'shock state' underlying the problem (see p. 295).

Type B lactic acidosis

Management of this type of acidosis involves the following.

(1) Investigation for any underlying conditions. Include a full blood count, electrolytes and urea, blood culture, blood glucose, serum amylase and calcium, ECG, microscopy and culture of urine and arterial blood gases. Blood should be taken for grouping, and serum saved for cross-matching. Unsuspected hypovolaemia may be revealed by a low CVP. A drug history may reveal that phenformin has been consumed.

(2) Treatment of the underlying condition is obviously of prime importance.

(3) Correction of the acidosis. Acidosis has a negative inotropic effect, and persistent acidosis will lead to shock and eventual death. It thus seems rational to treat the acidosis vigorously and early, in an attempt to halt this progression. Several measures have been advocated, although none has been subjected to controlled trial.

    (i) Infuse isotonic (1.26%) $NaHCO_3$ at a rate sufficient to bring the blood pH up to normal within 2–6 h, and then to keep it there. You will probably need between 600 mmol and 1500 mmol $NaHCO_3$ to achieve this.

    (ii) Methylene blue 5 mg/kg given as an infusion to buffer excess lactate.

    (iii) Haemodialysis and peritoneal dialysis have both been used, without any great enthusiasm or success.

    (iv) Dichloroacetate. This is a powerful activator of pyruvate dehydrogenase, and induces a striking decrease in lactate concentration. It should be given at a dose of 50 g/kg body weight, infused in 0.9 N saline (154 mmol/l) over 30 min.[6]

(4) Hypoxaemia should be corrected using 50–60% O_2 by face mask.

REFERENCES

(1) Alberti K. G. M. M., Nattrass M. (1977). Lactic acidosis. *Lancet*; **ii:** 25.

2   Bihari D. J. (1986). Metabolic acidosis. *Br. J. Hosp. Med.*; **35**: 89.

3   Gabow P. *et al.* (1980). Diagnostic importance of an increased
     serum anion gap. *N. Engl. J. Med.*; **303:** 854.
4   Gennari F. J. (1984). Serum osmolality. *N. Engl. J. Med.*; **310:**
     102.
5   Park R., Arieff A. I. (1983). Lactic acidosis—current concepts.
     Clin. Endocrinol. Metab.; **12**(2): 339.
6   Stackpoole P. W. *et al.* (1983). Treatment of lactic acidosis with
     dichloroacetate. *N. Engl. J. Med.*; **309:** 390.

Hypoglycaemic pre-coma and coma[1,2]

DIAGNOSIS

(1) Hypoglycaemia must be considered in any confused, disorientated, aggressive or excitable person, especially if he or she is known to be a diabetic on insulin, or taking sulphonylureas.

(2) Hypoglycaemia may be precipitated by alcohol, among other things. This mixture may be a difficult diagnostic problem to grapple with (sometimes literally) and is of medicolegal significance.

(3) Coma is an emergency par excellence.[2] Minutes count if irreversible brain damage is to be prevented. It is characterised by pallor, a moist skin, dilated pupils and possibly tachycardia.

(4) The significance of these signs may not strike the observer and hypoglycaemia must be considered and excluded in any unconscious patient. BM stix are adequate for this purpose and if they show a glucose content of less than 2.3 mmol/l (40 mg/100 ml), treatment should be given without waiting for the blood glucose result, for which blood should be taken first.

(5) The only thing that hypoglycaemic coma and hyperglycaemic coma have in common is that in both the patient may be diabetic and unconscious. BM stix reliably distinguish the two. If you are still doubtful, give dextrose i.v. (see below). It will do little harm to a patient in hyperglycaemic coma and will usually restore consciousness in patients with hypoglycaemic coma.

(6) Occasionally hypoglycaemia may present with focal neurological signs such as hemiplegia or focal fits (p. 198).

(7) **NEVER** give insulin as a 'diagnostic test' for a patient in coma In hypoglycaemia it is usually fatal and invariably disastrous.

MANAGEMENT

(1) Take blood for blood glucose, before initiating any treatment

(2) If the patient can drink, give 25 g dextrose in orange juice.

(3) If the patient is comatose, give 25 g dextrose i.v. (50 ml of 50% dextrose) and when the patient rouses, a further 25 g to drink

(4) Glucagon may be given in the following conditions.

(i)   If the patient cannot be restrained for long enough to give an i.v. injection safely, give glucagon 1 mg i.m., which raises blood sugar to within the normal range in 5–10 min, although its action is short-lived.

(ii)   Sulphonylureas reduce hepatic release of glucose, probably as a consequence of their effect on raising insulin levels. The insulin antagonist action of glucagon may help reverse this process, and so glucagon should be used in any patient whose hypoglycaemia is induced by sulphonylureas.

(5) Recovery is usually complete in 10–15 min but may take up to 1 h occasionally, despite adequate blood glucose levels.

(6) When the crisis is over, consider the cause.

(7) In patients rendered hypoglycaemic by long-acting insulins, or whom you suspect of taking really large doses of any insulin, after you have undertaken the initial therapy as outlined above, you should put up a 10% dextrose drip, and keep this running for at least 48 h. This is to forestall the real danger of hypoglycaemia recurring over the ensuing 24–48 h. The same strictures apply to hypoglycaemia induced by the sulphonylureas. The blood sugar, as monitored by BM stix, should be maintained between 5 mmol/l and 7 mmol/l.

(8) In any case, recovery of consciousness should be buttressed by a good meal.

REFERENCES

1   Jarrett R. J. (1971). Blood glucose homeostasis. *Br. J. Hosp. Med.*; **6:** 499.

2   Leader (1985). Hypoglycaemia and the nervous system. *Lancet*; **ii:** 759.

Addisonian crisis

Addisonian crisis may be primary, due to destruction or atrophy of the adrenal gland, or secondary, due to failure of the hypothalamic–pituitary–adrenal axis. The usual cause of secondary hypoadrenalism is the previous administration of exogenous steroids. Since, theoretically, only the glucocorticoid secretion is under pituitary control, mineralocorticoid deficiency should occur in primary but not in secondary hypoadrenalism. In fact, there is a tendency for the whole adrenal cortex to atrophy after long-term steroid ingestion, and mineralocorticoid deficiency may be assumed to be present in secondary hypoadrenalism.

DIAGNOSIS

(1) It should be considered in any hypotensive patient, who may also be vomiting, especially if they have received steroids within the past year. The signs of chronic adrenal insufficiency may or may not be present, so do not necessarily expect a pigmented, asthenic patient.

(2) It may be precipitated by infection, myocardial or cerebral infarction, trauma (including surgery), parturition or any metabolic stress. It may complicate septicaemia caused by pyogenic organisms—usually the *Meningococcus*—and is said to be due to haemorrhage into the adrenals. However, the majority of these patients are probably suffering from bacterial shock, for the plasma cortisols when measured are usually appropriately high.

(3) It is a useful, if cynical, maxim that in the above situation no one should be allowed to die with unexplained hypotension or coma without first receiving 200 mg of hydrocortisone i.v.

MANAGEMENT

The patient is depleted of sodium, potassium and water and may be hypoglycaemic. Take blood for baseline haemoglobin and PCV, electrolytes and urea, blood glucose and plasma cortisol and ACTH.

Arrange an abdominal x-ray, which may show adrenal calcification. Then manage as follows.

(1) Steroid replacement. Give 100 mg hydrocortisone sodium succinate i.v. and 100 mg i.m. and then 50 mg i.m. 8-hourly. Although hydrocortisone is essentially a glucocorticoid, it has sufficient mineralocorticoid activity when used in the above dosage to make it the drug of choice in both primary and secondary adrenal failure. However, some authorities suggest that a mineralocorticoid, such as deoxycorticosterone 10 mg i.m., should be given in any case where there is profound hypotension or clinical shock.

(2) Estimate blood glucose by BM stix. If less than 2.3 mmol/l (40 mg%), give 25 g of glucose orally or i.v. without waiting for the blood sugar results.

(3) Put up a drip, preferably with a CVP line. Give at least 1 litre of N saline in 2 h and then as necessary to keep the CVP within the normal range.

(4) Consider the cause.

(i) Do an ECG which may demonstrate myocardial infarction or hypokalaemia.

(ii) Look for signs of infection. Do not start a broad-spectrum antibiotic as routine. However, if the patient is pyrexial without obvious cause, investigations should include a chest x-ray, urine microscopy and blood cultures and then start on a broad-spectrum antibiotic parenterally. Bear in mind that hyperpyrexia does occur occasionally as a feature of Addisonian crisis.

(5) By now the electrolyte results should be available.

(i) Hyponatraemia needs further treatment with normal saline.

(ii) Potassium supplements may be necessary.

(iii) Further fluid replacement will depend on how much salt and water depletion has occurred. The commonest cause of continuing hypotension is hypovolaemia. Therefore, if in doubt, set up a CVP line and replace accordingly (see p. 343).

(6) Repeat the blood electrolytes 8-hourly if rapid fluid replacement is necessary. Water intoxication can easily occur in these patients if hypotonic saline is given, and the serum sodium should not be allowed to fall below 125 mmol/l.

Myxoedema coma[1,2]

DIAGNOSIS

(1) Patients usually present during the winter months, being particularly susceptible to hypothermia. It may, therefore, complicate conditions where hypothermia is common, such as strokes or chlorpromazine overdose.

(2) Before coma supervenes the patient may have been mentally dulled or psychotic.

(3) Usually the patient has the classical appearance and signs of myxoedema, except the delayed relaxation time of deep tendon reflexes which cannot be elicited. Hypotension and bradycardia are invariable.

(4) If coma has occurred, two-thirds of patients die. This may be due to insufficient appreciation of the multiple causes—2(i)–(vii) below—of coma.[3]

(5) Onset of coma may be accompanied by convulsions, which are treated in the usual way (see p. 210).

(6) It is, on occasions, difficult to know whether a patient in coma has myxoedema or not, especially as both thyroxine and tri-iodothyronine may be low in any very ill person. If you are in genuine doubt, it is worth treating as for myxoedema coma, as you are not likely to do any harm in the short term.

MANAGEMENT

(1) Measure blood glucose with BM stix and take blood for full blood count, electrolytes and urea, blood glucose, cortisol thyroxine or tri-iodothyronine and blood gases.

(2) Treat the following as indicated.

    (i)   Hypothyroidism. Whether to give l-triiodothyronine (T3) or thyroxine (T4) or both, and how much of each you should give is a subject steeped in controversy. The effect of T3 begins in 4 h or so, whereas T4 takes longer to act. However, T4 replacement is easier and more reliable, and its action is smoother. We think a reasonable policy is to give both, as outlined below.

(a) l-triiodothyronine (T3). Give 10 μg 6-hourly, either by nasogastric tube or i.v. if a suitable preparation is available.

(b) In addition, give T4 200 μg i.v. stat. and then 100 μg i.v. daily thereafter for two doses. The dosage of both the above should be halved if you are confident that your patient is suffering from ischaemic heart disease.

(ii) Hypoadrenalism. This will be present in all cases of myxoedema coma associated with hypopituitarism. As the pituitary status in any given patient with myxoedema coma may not be known, all should be given 100 mg hydrocortisone i.v. stat. and then 50 mg i.m. 8-hourly.

(iii) Hypoventilation. This may give rise to hypoxia alone or hypoxia and hypercarbia. Measure the blood gases. If the $Pa\text{CO}_2$ is raised (40 mmHg, 5.3 kPa) ventilation will be required; ventilation may also be required if the $Pa\text{O}_2$ cannot be kept above 60 mmHg (8.0 kPa) with O_2 via a face mask.

(iv) Hypothermia. Do not warm the patient rapidly. This may cause cardiovascular collapse. Simply use lots of blankets (see p. 265).

(v) Hypoglycaemia. If this is present, give 25 g of dextrose i.v. as frequently as necessary.

(vi) Hypotension. If the above measures do not restore the blood pressure, give plasma expanders—blood, Haemaccel, dextran 70 or plasma, whichever is available. If hypotension persists after hypovolaemia is corrected, as verified by a CVP line, it may be necessary to use an inotrope (see p. 16).

(vii) Hyponatraemia. This is nearly always caused by dilution and redistribution, possibly due to inappropriate ADH secretion. The appropriate treatment is fluid restriction. Attempts to correct hyponatraemia by hypertonic saline infusions merely exacerbate fluid retention. However, if the serum sodium is less than 120 mmol/l and the patient is now oedematous, it is possible that hyponatraemia may be contributory to the coma. In this situation give 50 ml increments of 5 N saline hourly (65 ml) and watch the CVP, lung bases and the effect on the serum sodium carefully.

REFERENCES

General reading

Belchetz P. E. (1984). Endocrine emergencies. In *Clinical Endocrinology.* (Keynes W., Fowler P. B., eds.). London: Heinemann Medical.

Hoffenberg R. (1980). Thyroid emergencies. *Clin. Endocrinol. Metab.*; **3:** 503.

Specific

1   Evered D., Hall R. (1972). Hypothyroidism. *Br. Med. J.*; **1:** 290.
2   Perlmutter M. (1964). Myxoedema crisis of pituitary or thyroid origin. *Am. J. Med.*; **36:** 883.
3   Royce P. C. (1971). Severely impaired consciousness in myxoedema. *Am. J. Med. Sci.*; **261:** 46.

Thyrotoxic crisis[3]

DIAGNOSIS

(1) The signs of breathlessness, anxiety, tremor, severe eyelid retraction and uncontrolled atrial fibrillation are virtually diagnostic. The thyroid gland is usually enlarged and obviously hyperactive, and the patient hyperpyrexial.

(2) However, patients can occasionally present with:

    (i)   a rapidly progressive weakness leading to drowsiness and coma;

    (ii)   an acute psychosis;

    (iii) abdominal pain and vomiting, simulating an acute abdominal crisis.

(3) It is usually precipitated by an infection, surgery, diabetic ketosis, or by prematurely stopping antithyroid treatment. It may occasionally occur following ^{131}I therapy for thyrotoxicosis, if the gland has not been suppressed beforehand with iodine.

MANAGEMENT

(1) Take blood for a full blood picture, electrolytes, blood glucose, and serum thyroxine, and save serum for tri-iodothyronine estimation should this be required later.

(2) Hyperthyroidism. Give:

    (i)   potassium iodide 600 mg i.v. over 1 h and then 2 g orally per day; this is reduced when the hyperthyroidism comes under control and its beneficial effect lasts not longer than 2 weeks;

    (ii)   propylthiouracil, 1000 mg/day, or carbimazole 100 mg/day by mouth (or stomach tube if necessary) in three divided doses. It is best to give the propylthiouracil 1 h before giving the potassium iodide, as this will ensure that the blockade of organification of iodine is established before the potassium iodide is given.

(3) Anxiety. If possible, the patient should be nursed by himself in a quiet semidark room.

    (i) Give chlorpromazine 100 mg i.v. This also helps treat hyperpyrexia.

    (ii) If anxiety is severe, an acute psychosis may supervene which, although sometimes resistant to chlorpromazine, usually responds to propranolol. The usual dose is 40 mg orally t.d.s., but it may be given i.v.—0.5–2 mg 6-hourly—if the patient is too sick to swallow. This may, however, precipitate severe hypotension and heart failure, and propranolol should not be used if there is pulmonary or peripheral oedema unless there is associated atrial fibrillation (see (4) below).[2] Start with the lower dose, increasing as necessary. Should heart failure supervene, atropine 0.4–1.0 mg i.v. should be given.

(4) Left ventricular failure.[4] This is caused by uncontrolled atrial fibrillation, which is treated along the usual lines with diuretics and oxygen (see p. 41). In addition propranolol, in the dosage described above, rapidly reduces the ventricular rate and restores sinus rhythm, thereby controlling the failure. Digoxin has no influence on the ventricular rate in this situation but is given as it increases the force of myocardial contraction. In atrial flutter, propranolol is theoretically dangerous.

(5) Hyperpyrexia. Some degree of fever is always present and does not necessarily indicate infection. Use fans, and tepid sponge together with chlorpromazine as above. Aspirin increases the metabolic rate, displaces thyroxine from prealbumin, and should not be used. If the above measures are ineffective propranolol given as above may cause dramatic improvement.

(6) Dehydration. This may occur from hyperventilation and sweating as well as insufficient fluid intake. CVP recordings are especially valuable in this situation as hypovolaemia may be complicated by heart failure. Give 20% or 33% dextrose i.v. as extra calories are needed to supply increased metabolic demands. In addition, cautious replacement of sodium losses will also be necessary. Do not attempt to raise the serum sodium by giving hypertonic saline as this may precipitate pulmonary oedema. Repeat the electrolytes after 12 h.

(7) Adrenal insufficiency. Hypotension and vomiting may be due to adrenocortical insufficiency which is unmasked by the

metabolic stress. Take blood for plasma cortisol and give 100 mg of hydrocortisone i.v. without waiting for the result, followed by 50 mg 6-hourly.

(8) Hypoxia. Occasional patients have a severe associated myopathy. This may give rise to ventilatory failure (see p. 67), so monitor the blood gases, and be prepared to institute IPPR as necessary.

(9) Thromboembolic complications. These appear to be common, and serious. Give heparin (see p. 17).

(10) Thyrotoxic crisis may be fatal and in severe cases it may be necessary to anaesthetise, paralyse and ventilate the patient in an attempt to reduce metabolic requirements.

(11) The use of haemoperfusion over a polyacrylamide gel column has been advocated in intractable thyrotoxic crisis. This technique looks promising and is worth considering.[1]

Effective therapy of the precipitating cause is a major determinant of the ultimate outcome.

REFERENCES

General reading
(See p. 178.)

Specific

1   Herrman J., Ruddorff K. H., Gockenjan G. (1977). Charcoal haemoperfusion in thyroid storm. *Lancet*; **i:** 248.

2   Ikram H. (1977). Haemodynamic effects of beta-adrenergic blockade in hyperthyroid patients with and without heart failure. *Br. Med. J.*; **1:** 1505.

3   Mackin J. F., Canary J. J., Pittmann C. S. (1974). Thyroid storm and its management. *N. Engl. J. Med.*; **291:** 1396

4   Skelton C. L. (1982). The heart in hyperthyroidism. *N. Engl. J. Med.*; **307:** 1206.

Acute hypercalcaemia[1,3,5]

This may be caused by hyperparathyroidism, vitamin D intoxication, widespread bone metastases,[6] non-metastatic complications of malignancies, the milk-alkali syndrome, myeloma or sarcoidosis (for differentiation see reference 2).

DIAGNOSIS

Polydipsia, polyuria, abdominal pain, disorders of behaviour, profound muscle weakness, vomiting and pyrexia may progress to cardiovascular collapse and coma. The inevitable fluid loss is accompanied by the loss of both magnesium and potassium. Acute renal failure, due in part to this hypovolaemia, may occur. A fatal cardiac arrhythmia may terminate the condition. The serum calcium in these cases is usually more than 4 mmol/l (16 mg/100 ml).

Conjunctivitis due to local calcific deposits on the corneoscleral junction is a most striking physical sign. It is best seen with a hand lens and strong lateral lighting. The ECG shows a shortened QT interval.

MANAGEMENT

(1) Take blood for haemoglobin, PCV, electrolytes (including Cl^- and Mg^{2+}) and urea, serum calcium, phosphate and alkaline phosphatase and plasma proteins.
(2) Rehydration. This is the single most important measure in the treatment of hypercalcaemia. Rehydrate your patient with isotonic saline and 5% dextrose, giving potassium and magnesium supplements as necessary—a CVP line is valuable. You may need 4–5 litres of N saline in the first 24 h. It is wise to add 20 mEq of K^+ and 10 mEq of Mg^{2+} to each litre, and monitor both K^+ and Mg^{2+}. This rehydration will invariably lower the serum Ca^{2+}, and may be the only treatment necessary.
(3) If the patient remains symptomatic, or the serum Ca^{2+} remains >3 mmol/l, you will need to lower the Ca^{2+} further. There are several ways of doing this, shown below in order of preference.

(i)   Frusemide 100 mg/h, in order to maintain a urine output of around 500 ml/h. This reduces the serum Ca^{2+} by a mean value of 0.75 mmol/l (3.1 mg/ml) over 24 h.

   The considerable fluid, Na^+, K^+ and Mg^{2+} losses should be measured frequently and replaced. This requires intensive care, but provided adequate attention is paid to correcting the fluid and electrolyte loss, it is a safe and effective way of lowering Ca^{2+}.

(ii)   Mithramycin 25 µg/kg i.v. over 3 h in a solution of 5% dextrose or by a bolus. This is usually effective within 12–36 h.

(iii)   A traditional but inconvenient method has been to use a solution of sodium phosphate buffer, pH 7.4 (81 mmol Na_2HPO_4 and 19 mmol NaH_2PO_4 made up to 1 litre with 19 mmol KCl added). The solution should be infused over 8 h, and has its maximum effect between 14 and 20 h. The amount you give can be assessed from the following data.

   (a) 100 mmol sodium phosphate (i.e. 1 litre of solution) infused over 8 h gives a mean Ca^{2+} depression of 1.5 mmol/l (6.1 mg/100 ml).

   (b) 75 mmol sodium phosphate infused over 8 h gives a mean serum Ca^{2+} depression of 1 mmol/l (4.1 mg/100 ml).

   (c) 50 mmol sodium phosphate infused over 8 h gives a mean serum Ca^{2+} depression of 0.6 mmol/l (2.4 mg/100 ml).

   The only problem with using phosphate solution is the tendency to precipitate calcium phosphate in the tissues. For this reason we would now suggest using either frusemide or mithramycin as the first line therapy (see above).

(iv)   If the patient has renal or cardiac failure, the volume of fluid and sodium load of this phosphate solution may be prohibitive and either mithramycin or dialysis (either peritoneal or haemo) against a calcium-free dialysate should be undertaken.[4]

As alternatives to the above treatments, the following have been used.

(v)   Calcitonin, which can be used in a dose of 8 units/kg i.m. 6-hourly, preferably as gelatin-based porcine calcitonin.

(vi) If the situation is not critical, phosphate (Na_2HPO_4 or K_2HPO_4) 1–4 g/day may be given orally.

(vii) Diphosphonates. These agents are potent inhibitors of osteoclastic bone resorption. Three drugs, sodium etidronate, clodronate disodium and aminohydroxypropylidene, have been used i.v. on a trial basis in the hypercalcaemia of malignancy. The results are encouraging, and when these drugs are generally available they are likely to become of increasing importance.

(4) As soon as the cause of the hypercalcaemia has been identified,[1,2] specific treatment should be started.

REFERENCES

1 Elliott G. T., McKenzie M. W. (1983). Treatment of hypercalcaemia: *Drug Intell. Clin. Pharmacol.*; **17:** 12.
2 Fraser P., Watson L., Healy M. (1976). Further experience with discriminant function in the differential diagnosis of hypercalcaemia. *Postgrad. Med. J.*; **52:** 254.
3 Fulmer D. H., Dimich A. B., Rothschild E. O. *et al.* (1972) Treatment of hypercalcaemia. *Arch. Intern. Med.*; **129:** 923.
4 Nolph K. D., Stoctz M., Maher J. F., (1971). Calcium free peritoneal dialysis. *Arch. Intern. Med.*; **128:** 809.
5 Stevenson J. C. (1985). Malignant hypercalcaemia. *Br. Med. J.*; **291:** 421.
6 Wilkinson R. (1984). Treatment of hypercalcaemia associated with malignancy. *Br. Med. J.*; **288:** 812.

Tetany

DIAGNOSIS

(1) This is usually diagnosed by observing the characteristic carpo-pedal spasm of the hands (and sometimes feet). This is usually heralded by circumoral paraesthesiae and may be accompanied by excessive neuromuscular irritability (the basis of Chvostek's sign).

(2) It is less easily recognised when it presents itself as laryngo-spasm, psychosis or generalised convulsions. Carpopedal spasm usually accompanies these manifestations but, if not, can usually be elicited by inflating a sphygmomanometer cuff above the systolic arterial pressure for 1 min.

CAUSES AND MANAGEMENT

(1) Hypocalcaemia. This occurs after parathyroid surgery, fol-lowing a prolonged 'forced' diuresis, in malabsorption and in rickets and osteomalacia, sometimes immediately after vitamin D therapy is started. If it is unrelieved, laryngeal spasm and generalised convulsions ensue. Psychotic behaviour may be prominent. Give 10% calcium gluconate i.v.; 20 ml of 10% calcium gluconate contains 176 mg of Ca^{2+}, and you usually require 15 mg Ca^{2+}/kg body weight. Give 20 ml in the first 10 min, and the rest by slow infusion over the next 12 h. Con-tinue with dihydrotachysterol, 3–10 ml (0.25 mg/ml) per day initially but reducing rapidly. Monitor the serum Ca^{2+} and PO_4^{2-}.

(2) Hyperventilation (see p. 335).

(3) Hypomagnesaemia. This can also cause a positive Chvostek's sign and convulsions. Give 5–40 mmol magnesium sulphate or chloride slowly i.v. (1 mmol of magnesium chloride hexa-hydrate = 200 mg; 1 mmol of magnesium sulphate = 246 mg).

(4) States of alkalotic hypokalaemia. These are usually seen when dehydration caused by vomiting is 'corrected' with infusions containing bicarbonate or lactate. Treatment is along the usual lines, with potassium supplements plus i.v. calcium gluconate as above.

(5) Rapid correction of chronic acidosis causes a decrease in ionised calcium and hence tetany. This is treated by giving calcium as in (1) above.

Section VI

Neurological

The completed stroke[14]

DIAGNOSIS

This usually presents itself as a sudden neurological deficit in a person who may have pre-existing arterial disease. In addition there may be loss of consciousness.

Strokes may be due to any of the following.

(1) Cerebral infarction (80% of strokes in most series.) The vessels may be occluded by thrombosis in situ, or by embolic material[13] arising from the following.

    (i)   The heart. Embolism is said rarely to be due to fibrillation alone unless the mitral valve is abnormal or the left atrium enlarged. Emboli arise from infected or calcified heart valves or from a prolapsing mitral valve.[11] Mural thrombi associated with myocardial infarction may become detached. Emboli from these sites may occlude vessels elsewhere and peripheral pulses must be checked.

    (ii)   Neck vessels, commonly from atheromatous plaques at the origin of the internal carotid artery. A bruit may be heard but if stenosis is tight, a bruit may be absent or contralateral.[1]

    (iii)   Thrombosis in situ. This usually occurs on atheromatous sections of the intracranial vessels. Thrombosis accounts for most internal capsular infarcts and also for most brainstem strokes, where occlusion of small end-vessels causes ischaemic scars (lacunae—so called because they look like small black dots at post mortem). Lacunae, 70% of which are associated with hypertension, may cause a wide variety of syndromes but may recognisably present as:[5,6]

        (a) pure motor stroke;
        (b) pure sensory stroke;
        (c) dysarthria with a clumsy hand;
        (d) ipsilateral ataxia with weakness of the leg.

Cerebral infarction secondary to thrombosis is not always caused by atheromatous disease; other causes such as arteritis (collagen

189

disease), syphilis, the contraceptive pill and polycythemia[19] should be excluded.

In all forms of infarction aside from lacunes, premonitory episodes of neurological deficit are not uncommon, meningism is rare, the CSF is not usually xanthochromic and, unless there is massive infarction, there is no shift of midline structures within the first 24 h. These features help to distinguish infarction from haemorrhage, a distinction which can only be reliably confirmed by a CT scan. However, a recent study has further refined our ability to distinguish clinically between the types of stroke using a score derived from eight clinical features.[2]

(2) Cerebral haemorrhage (15% of strokes; the residual 5% are patients who present as strokes, but turn out to have other lesions).[12] The haemorrhage may be primarily intracerebral or subarachnoid.

   (i) Primarily intracerebral. Bleeding in people with hypertension usually occurs from minute, thin-walled aneurysmal dilatation of intracranial arteries—Charcot–Bouchard aneurysms. Occasionally, bleeding occurs from vascular malformations in normotensive patients. In about three-quarters of cases the bleeding spreads from the brain substance into the subarachnoid space and the resulting meningeal irritation gives rise to vomiting, headache and neck stiffness. Within the first 24 h the haematoma, in about three-quarters of cases, causes a shift of midline structures (as identified by echoencephalography or by the position of the calcified pineal on an AP skull x-ray). CT scan reliably detects haemorrhage and, if this is readily available, lumbar puncture should not be performed because of the slight risk of coning. If CT scan is not available, a lumbar puncture is still the best way of confirming haemorrhage, although the CSF is normal in 45% of patients with haemorrhage proven by CT scan.

   (ii) Primarily subarachnoid.[4,9] The bleeding occurs from an aneurysm (65%) or AV malformation (5%) directly into the subarachnoid space. In 20%, no cause is found, and in these cases the prognosis is good.[18] The symptoms, which characteristically start abruptly, are those of meningeal irritation, with or without loss of consciousness. Focal neurological deficits may be present due to arterial spasm or extension of haemorrhage into the brain. The combination of a focal neurological deficit in a patient with signs of subacute bacterial endocarditis strongly suggest mycotic aneurysm. Blood in the subarachnoid space may be identified by CT scan and if so lumbar puncture is unnecessary.

If the CT scan is unavailable or unrevealing, a lumbar puncture should be carried out—remember that occasionally an early lumbar puncture will show normal CSF since it make take 24 h for blood to appear in the lumbar CSF. All bloody CSF should be centrifuged so that subarachnoid bleeding, identified by the xanthochromic supernatant, may be distinguished from a traumatic tap where the supernatant is clear. When a subarachnoid haemorrhage has been identified, the timing of four-vessel arteriography should be discussed with your neurosurgical colleagues. Other therapeutic interventions which have been advocated are discussed later (see p. 194).

In any unconscious patient other causes of unconsciousness must be excluded (see p. 323). In addition, the following conditions may cause diagnostic confusion.[15]

(1) Subdural haematoma. A history of head injury, while typical, may be lacking, especially in patients with pre-existing cortical atrophy. Percussion of the skull may reveal lateralised tenderness sufficient to arouse deeply stuporous patients, and also an area of dullness over the haematoma.[8]

Inequality of the pupils and a fluctuating but overall deteriorating level of consciousness, with progressive focal neurological signs, are all highly suggestive.

There may be a shift of midline structures and the diagnosis may be confirmed with CT scan. However, if subdural haematomas are bilateral, there may be no mass effect, and if isodense, may be undetectable on CT scan. The very normality of the CT scan in a clearly deteriorating patient is in itself suspicious, and the diagnosis may be made by a radionuclide brain scan or, if necessary, arteriography.

(2) Extradural haematoma.

(3) Brain tumour: 3–5% of clinically diagnosed acute strokes turn out to be due to a tumour. Calcification may be present on skull x-ray or CT scan. Arteriography may reveal neovascularisation.

(4) Brain abscess. This usually occurs in the setting of purulent lung

disease, infected ears or nasal sinuses, or in patients with a right-to-left intracardiac shunt. Ring enhancement is typically seen on CT scan but may be difficult to distinguish from a brain tumour.

(5) As we have suggested earlier, the differentiation from strokes of the mass lesions described in (1)–(4) above can only be made confidently with a CT scan. CT scans are not everywhere readily available, but in any 'stroke' patient with:

(i) a history on admission suggestive of a gradually evolving focal deficit, particularly if the progression has been in a continuous rather than stepwise fashion,

(ii) a clear history of either generalised or focal fits,

(iii) a deficit which clearly worsens in the 24 h after admission, you should consider the desirability of obtaining a scan.[16]

(6) Hemiplegic migraine. A history of preceding or accompanying visual disturbance, a throbbing headache which is associated with nausea, and photophobia, usually in a young person in association with a normal CSF, clinches the diagnosis.

(7) Epileptic attacks, particularly those associated with residual paralysis (Todd's paralysis), may also temporarily be mistaken for strokes.

MANAGEMENT

The main purpose of the investigation is to determine if any treatable causes (see below), unfortunately the minority, are present. The history and clinical findings may help.

(1) The investigation of choice is a CT scan. This will, with a high degree of reliability, distinguish between a stroke and other lesions, as well as between haemorrhagic and other types of stroke.[16] It is clearly impractical, and anyway not good medicine, to obtain a CT scan on all patients. Fortunately, there are now reasonable guidelines on which to act, which have been outlined in (5) above. The other circumstances in which we recommend obtaining a CT scan are:

(a) if you are contemplating anticoagulant or antiplatelet therapy, as you need to ensure that the lesion is not haemorrhagic (see section 3 p. 199); and

(b) if you have diagnosed a cerebellar lesion, as surgery may be helpful here (see section 2 p. 194).[17]

(2) The skull x-ray still has a place and should be done particularly if there is any question of head injury.
(3) If subarachnoid haemorrhage is suspected, CT examination is the investigation of choice. If this facility is not available, CSF examination should be undertaken, but is, of course, contra-indicated where there are signs or symptoms of raised intra-cranial pressure.
(4) Arteriography may be required to localise the space-occupying lesion if a CT scan is not available, and is anyway indicated in the further investigation of subarachnoid haemorrhage.

Full blood picture and ESR, VDRL and FTA–ABS may detect the rare cases of collagen disease, syphilis or polycythaemia which are treated on their merits.

General measures

(1) General care of the helpless and/or comatose patient (see p. 322).
(2) Treatment of complications which may follow a stroke.

   (i)   Dehydration. This is avoided by feeding fluids through a nasogastric tube if the patient has a cough reflex, and if not, by giving fluids i.v.
   (ii) Hypothermia (see p. 265).
   (iii) Hyperthermia (temperature >40°C (104°F)). This usually occurs in conjunction with a pontine lesion. If severe it may itself cause depression of consciousness; consequently, cooling the patient with tepid sponging is occasionally associated with marked improvement.
   (iv) Diabetes. This may be precipitated by an intracranial catastrophe. However, the transient glycosuria which may follow a stroke needs no treatment unless ketosis occurs.
   (v)   Fits. These need treatment in the usual way (see p. 210).
   (vi) Hypertension. This may be a transient phenomenon, set-tling within a few hours of the stroke. If it persists (i.e. a diastolic pressure above 120 mmHg), it would seem logical to reduce this to a level appropriate to the patient's age. However, following a stroke, the autoregulatory capacity of blood vessels in the brain may be impaired for a period of about 3 weeks. This means that, in contradis-tinction to normal, the flow in the diseased area becomes

pressure dependent. Lowering arterial pressure will thus reduce flow to this area. Against this is the danger of continuing hypertension damaging residual healthy brain. We advocate, as a compromise, gentle reduction of arterial pressure until the diastolic is less than 110 mmHg and the systolic less than 170 mmHg. This should be accomplished where possible by conventional oral hypotensive therapy. Failing this, hydralazine, initially 10 mg i.m., is a reasonable drug to use.

(vii) Hypertensive encephalopathy. The considerations in (vi) above do not apply if there is evidence of hypertensive encephalopathy (see p. 44).

(viii) Cerebral oedema. Seen as low attenuation with mass effect on CT scan, it reflects the volume of ischaemic tissue. It may occasionally cause papilloedema. There is no evidence that dexamethasone affects the oedema surrounding infarction or that it alters the mortality or morbidity following stroke. Dexamethasone is, however, extremely effective in reducing oedema surrounding tumour or abscess and may be given as 6 mg 6-hourly.[7] An acute rise in intracranial pressure may be treated by a bolus of 20% mannitol 1–2 g/kg i.v. over 5–10 min.

Specific measures

In general, determining the cause of a completed stroke has little immediate therapeutic spin-off. However, in the following situations specific therapy may be helpful.

(1) Primary subarachnoid haemorrhage (see above). There is real danger of re-bleeding in this group, and neurosurgical advice should be sought when the diagnosis is made. Early treatment with an antifibrinolytic agent such as epsilon aminocaproic acid (EACA) 24 g orally per day, or tranexamic acid, has not been found to be helpful.[20] However, it seems that the calcium antagonists may be helpful, and some now give nimodipine 0.7 mg/kg as an initial dose, then 0.35 mg/kg 4-hourly.[3,10] Beta-blockers are also said to be helpful.[21] We remain to be convinced. Surgery to prevent re-bleeding should always be considered in this group, particularly in the patient with little neurological impairment (see p. 190).

(2) Cerebellar haematoma. This merits separate mention as it is

amenable to surgery. Unfortunately, progression to coma and death is rapid due to brainstem compression. In the short interval before coma the patient may complain of occipital headache and vertigo. There is a gaze palsy to the side of the haemorrhage. Mild ipsilateral peripheral VIIth nerve palsy and dysarthria are common, but only a minority show nystagmus or ipsilateral ataxia. Contralateral hemiplegia does not occur, so the finding of a gaze palsy without limb paralysis is a useful pointer. Diagnosis is by CT scan.

(3) Embolism. The diagnosis of embolism rests on the acute onset of neurological deficit in a patient with a source of emboli, e.g. atrial fibrillation. Further emboli may be prevented by adequate and early anticoagulation.[13] However, up to 30% of infarcts secondary to embolism and haemorrhagic, as demonstrated on CT scan or by the presence of blood or xanthochromia in the CSF. Early anticoagulation in this group may precipitate disastrous secondary haemorrhage and should be delayed for approximately 2 weeks. It follows from the above that, wherever possible, you must get an urgent CT scan before starting a course of anticoagulants.

(4) When any of the causes considered under differential diagnosis are found, appropriate therapy should be instituted.

REFERENCES

1   Ackerman R. H. (1979). Perspective of non-invasive diagnosis of carotid disease. *Neurology (Minneap.)*; **29:** 615.

2   Allen C. M. C. (1983). Clinical diagnosis of the acute stroke syndrome. *Quart. J. Med.*; **42:** 515.

3   Allen G. S. (1983). Cerebral arterial spasm. A controlled trial of nifedipine in patients with sub-arachnoid haemorrhage. *N. Engl. J. Med.*; **308:** 619.

4   Bartlett J. R. (1981). Subarachnoid haemorrhage. *Br. Med. J.*; **283:** 1347.

5   Critchley E. M. R. (1983). Recognition and management of lacunar strokes. *Br. Med. J.*; **287:** 777.

6   Fisher C. M. (1965). Lacunes: small deep cerebral infarcts. *Neurology (Minneap.)*; **15:** 774.

7   Fishman R. A. (1982). Steroids in brain oedema. *N. Engl. J. Med.*; **306:** 359.

8   Guarino J. R. (1981). Auscultatory percussion of the head. *Br. Med. J.*; **1:** 1075.

9   Hitchcock E. R. (1983). Ruptured aneurysms. *Br. Med. J.*; **286:** 1299.
10 Leader (1983). Calcium antagonists and aneurysmal subarachnoid haemorrhage. *Lancet*; **ii:** 141.
11 Leader (1981). Mitral valve prolapse. *Br. Med. J.*; **282:** 1411.
12 Leader (1984). Stroke: was it haemorrhage or infarct? *Lancet*; **i:** 204.
13 Leader (1985). Cerebral embolism. *Lancet*; **i:** 29.
14 Management of stroke (1985). *Drugs. Therap. Bull.*; **23:** 9.
15 Norris J. W., Hachinski V. C. (1982). Misdiagnosis of a stroke. *Lancet*; **i:** 328.
16 Sandercock P. *et al.* (1985). Value of computed tomography in patients with stroke. *Br. Med. J.*; **290:** 193.
17 Shenkin H. A. (1982). Cerebellar strokes. *Lancet*; **ii:** 479.
18 Shepard R. H. (1984). Prognosis of spontaneous subarachnoid haemorrhage of unknown cause. *Lancet*; **i:** 777.
19 Thomas D. J., Marshall J., Ross Russell R. W. (1977). Effect of haematocrit on cerebral blood flow in man. *Lancet*; **ii:** 941.
20 Vermeulen M. *et al.* (1984). Antifibrinolytic treatment in subarachnoid haemorrhage. *N. Engl. J. Med.*; **311:** 432.
21 Walter P. *et al.* (1982). Beneficial effect of adrenergic blockade in patients with subarachnoid haemorrhage. *Br. Med. J.*; **284:** 1661.

Transient ischaemic attacks (TIAs)[3,5,10]

DIAGNOSIS

These are episodes of transient neurological deficit. They may be recurrent, sometimes only last a few minutes, and are due to temporary reduction in blood supply to part of the brain. The importance of recognising TIAs is that they are followed by major stroke with a frequency of about 5% per annum, particularly if the TIA is in the carotid territory.

They may be due to the following causes.

(1) Emboli arising from atheroma of the vertebral and carotid arteries, or their branches, or from the heart. This is the single most important cause of TIA.[1,11]

(2) In the setting of borderline local cerebral perfusion, transient reduction in overall cerebral blood flow may cause significant, albeit temporary, local ischaemia. This can occur on the basis of:

    (i)   a fall in perfusion pressure due to:

        (a) hypotension e.g. hypotensive drugs (see p. 45),
        (b) decreased cardiac output (e.g. arrhythmias);[7]

    (ii)   increased viscosity due to:

        (a) a PCV of above 50%,
        (b) paraproteinaemia.

(3) Transient reduction in local blood flow, which may be the result of any of the following.

    (i)   Hypertension. Focal neurological deficit may occur as part of hypertensive encephalopathy (see p. 44).

    (ii)   Migraine. Complicated migraine may occasionally cause hemiplegia characterised more by dysaesthesiae than weakness, or a third or sixth nerve palsy (ophthalmoplegic migraine). It is usually possible to elicit a history of previous attacks of 'classical' migraine.

    (iii) Mechanical effects on flow.

        (a) Neck movements may cause occlusion of the vertebral arteries with ensuing posterior cerebral and brainstem ischaemia. Failure of autoregulation of the

posterior cerebral circulation may cause the structures so supplied to be vulnerable to changes of the
systemic circulation. This may play a role in 'vertebral basilar insufficiency'.

(b) Subclavian steal. In this condition, movement of the
arms diverts blood from the vertebral arteries causing
symptoms of transient brainstem ischaemia.

(4) Lack of nutrients, which presumably cause focal symptoms on
the same basis as (2) above.

(i) Anaemia. Haemoglobin of less than 7 g/100 ml may be
the sole cause of TIA.

(ii) Hypoglycaemia. This may rarely present itself with a
focal neurological deficit.

In a proportion of cases no cause can be found, presumably
because of lysis of the vascular obstruction, or because the vessel
involved is too small to be identified.

(5) TIAs should be differentiated from:

(i) focal epilepsy: in focal epilepsy, the patient often complains of positive symptoms (e.g. paraesthesiae, spontaneous movements); these are uncommon in TIAs;

(ii) Todd's paralysis: this is the transient focal weakness that
occurs after an epileptic seizure.

(6) Attacks resembling TIAs may be the initial symptoms of cerebral tumours. These are presumably caused by alteration of
circulation in the adjacent brain.

Examination therefore must include careful auscultation of the
head, heart and neck, measurement of lying and standing arterial
pressure and the pressure in each arm, and assessment of peripheral
vasculature. A 24 h continuous ECG, plasma glucose, lipid profile
and cholesterol and full blood picture and ESR may establish an
underlying cause which should be dealt with accordingly. A prolap-
sing leaflet of the mitral valve may give rise to a loud midsystolic click
or be silent, and can be confirmed with echocardiography.[6]

MANAGEMENT

There are several uncontroversial aspects of management, including
the following.

(1) Control of hypertension. The diastolic pressure should be slowly reduced to less than 100 mmHg. Thiazide diuretics and propranolol are useful hypotensive agents as they minimise the chances of postural hypotension. Reduction of arterial pressure may be all that is required to control TIA.

(2) Control of blood glucose.

(3) Reduction of PCV to below 45% by repeated small (200 ml) venesections.

(4) Reduction of hypercholesterolaemia or hyperlipidaemia, and the control of other risk factors, such as smoking.

(5) Prophylactic anticoagulants following emboli arising from the heart (see p. 195).

(6) The control of any cardiac arrhythmia.

There are three other modes of therapy; each has its proponents.

(1) Endarterectomy.[9]

(2) Prophylactic anticoagulants.

(3) Inhibition of platelet function with aspirin 150–300 mg daily.[2,6,8] The addition of other antiplatelet agents does not help.

It is possible that TIA due to atheromatous disease of the cerebral blood vessels has several causes, and that different subgroups of patients are affected (favourably or adversely) by these methods of treatment. Well-controlled trials of each against no treatment are rare, and those against each other are in progress.

In our current ignorance, one accepted course of practice is to perform four-vessel arteriography (preferably with a digital vascular imager[5]) in patients who are otherwise surgically acceptable and in whom no other cause has been found (see above), and to operate on significant stenosis or deeply ulcerated plaques detected in the carotid system.

Anticoagulants may be used in patients with intrinsic carotid disease where no operable lesion is identified, who have no medical contraindication, who are judged to take medicines reliably, and who can be closely supervised. Aspirin may be used in the remainder. It should be remembered, however, that the major cause of death in patients with TIAs, is cardiovascular disease and that treatment directed solely to the cerebral circulation may be irrelevant to the patient as a whole.

REFERENCES

1   De Bono D. P., Warlow C. P. (1981). Potential sources of emboli in patients with presumed TIAs. *Lancet*; **i:** 343.

2   Fields L. S. (1983). Aspirin for prevention of stroke: a review. *Am. J. Med.*; **74:** 63.

3   Kistler J. P. *et al.* (1984). Therapy of ischaemic cerebrovascular disease due to atherothrombosis. *N. Engl. J. Med.*; **311:** 27.

4   Leader (1982). Amaurosis fugax. *Lancet*; **i:** 838.

5   Leader (1985). Computerised intravenous arteriography. *Lancet*; **ii:** 813.

6   Leader (1986). Aspirin: what dose? *Lancet*; **i:** 592.

7   McAllen P. M., Marshall J. (1973). Cardiac dysrhythmia and transient cerebral ischaemic attacks. *Lancet*; **i:** 1212.

8   Marcus A. J. (1983). Aspirin as an antithrombotic medication. *N. Engl. J. Med.*; **309:** 1515.

9   Warlow C. P. (1984). Carotid endarterectomy: does it work? *Stroke*; **15:** 1068.

10 Warlow C. P. (1985). Transient ischaemic attacks. Current treatment concepts. *Drugs*; **29:** 474.

11 Wynne J. (1986). Mitral valve prolapse. *N. Engl. J. Med.*; **314** 577.

Closed head injury[4,5,7]

DIAGNOSIS

(1) This is not usually in doubt, but needs to be considered with every unconscious patient. Witnesses should be sought.

(2) It may be suggested by careful examination of the head and neck. Blood and/or CSF in the external auditory canal or behind the tympanic membrane indicates a basal skull fracture. An anterior fossa fracture may be indicated by CSF rhinorrhoea or periorbital haematomata. Vitreous haemorrhage may occur following a whiplash injury, particularly in children.

(3) It may occur in the setting of other conditions, some of which may also cause coma, for example acute alcoholic intoxication. In this situation, as in all cases of coma with suspected head injury, the skull should be x-rayed. A skull fracture cannot be diagnosed clinically, is a strong indication of the severity of the injury, and may therefore be associated with intracranial pathology which may only become apparent after an interval.

(4) Consideration should be given to injury elsewhere, particularly in the neck (see p. 202).

MANAGEMENT

Head injuries may give rise to unconsciousness and death because of the contusion and haemorrhage sustained at the time. Frequently, however, it is events subsequent to the injury which account for considerable morbidity and mortality. The major part of this is the development of cerebral oedema, which in turn compromises cerebral blood flow. This cerebral oedema is in part a consequence of the primary brain injury, but is frequently compounded by extracranial, and potentially reversible, factors such as hypoxia, hypotension usually secondary to hypovolaemia, fits and infection. Due attention must be given to these secondary events, which do not themselves require special neurosurgical expertise, but are at least as important as the consequences of the primary injury.[6]

Therefore management should include the following steps, in approximate order of priority.

(1) Check the airway. If ventilation is in doubt, either because of brainstem involvement or for peripheral reasons (inhaled blood or vomit or chest injury), intubate and ventilate.

(2) Check the arterial pressure. Hypotension usually results from blood loss from injuries elsewhere,[1] but occurs occasionally for central reasons. Treatment is along the usual lines, with volume (usually blood) replacement and pressor agents if necessary (see p. 298).

(3) Control fits, if any (p. 210).

(4) Examine the neck. If there is local pain, evidence of trauma or evidence of loss of power or sensation in the limbs, do not move the patient until a lateral neck x-ray has been obtained.

(5) Do not give opiates for pain, phenobarbitone for restlessness or mydriatics for convenient observation of the fundi, since interpretation of the pupillary response is extremely important.

(6) When the ventilation, circulation and fits are satisfactorily controlled, assess the level of consciousness. We recommend the use of the Glasgow coma, or more correctly, consciousness scale. Three elements of behaviour are scored.

(i) Eye opening.

Response	Score
Nil	1 (no response to any stimulus)
Pain	2 (infraorbital pressure)
Verbal	3 (response to a loud command)
Spontaneous (with blinking)	4

(ii) Motor response (to infraorbital pressure).

Response	Score
Nil	1
Abnormal extension	2 (extension of both arms and legs)
Abnormal flexion	3 (flexion preceded by extension)
Weak flexion	4 (flexor withdrawal response)
Localising	5 (able to use a limb to locate and resist the noxious stimulus)
Obeys commands	6

(The arms are usually more responsive than the legs; in the case of different patterns in arms and legs, always record the best response.)

(iii) Verbal response.

Response	Score	
Nil	1	
Incomprehensible	2	(mumbling—no recognisable words)
Inappropriate	3	(intelligible, isolated words—often profanities —no phrases)
Confused	4	(correct phrases, but disorientated and confused in context)
Fully orientated	5	

Information derived from these observations should be recorded on a chart. Deterioration in the level of consciousness implies progression of the neuronal damage. This calls for an urgent reappraisal of the situation, usually by a more experienced colleague (see below).

(7) Now that most doctors are aware of the importance of the general supportive measures outlined above, improvement in the outcome of head-injured patients will depend on the early recognition and treatment of focal intracranial haemorrhage.[3,8] Unfortunately, the traditional diagnostic pointers appear late, so the central issue with which you have to grapple is: which head-injured patients require a CT scan? Dispute about this naturally rages, but fortunately there are now reasonable guidelines.

You should consult your neurosurgical colleagues, with a view to getting both advice and a CT scan, if your patient has had any of the following.

(i) A fractured skull associated with any of the following:

(a) any impairment of consciousness,
(b) one or more fits,
(c) any other neurological symptoms or signs.

(ii) Coma which persists after resuscitation, even if there is no skull fracture.

(iii) Any deterioration in the level of consciousness, as assessed by the Glasgow coma scale.

- (iv) Any neurological disturbance which persists for 8 h after resuscitation, even if there is no skull fracture.
- (v)   A depressed fracture of the skull vault.
- (vi) Any suspicion of a fracture of the base of the skull.

Further management

Bearing all this in mind, we can categorise patients with significant head injuries into one of three groups.

Group 1: Spontaneous improvement (the majority). These patients need careful observation in hospital and, if all is well (see (8) above), can usually be discharged 24 h after they have fully recovered. Careful observation should consist for at least 6 h of ¼-hourly recording and charting of the following.

- (i)   Pulse.
- (ii) Arterial pressure.

      Charting of these allows the trend to be recognised if the pulse is slowing or arterial pressure rising in the case of increasing intracranial pressure; similarly, a rising pulse and falling arterial pressure will indicate occult haemorrhage.

- (iii) Respiration. An altered ventilatory pattern (and/or depth) may indicate brainstem compromise (p. 317).
- (iv) Conscious level (see above).
- (v)   Pupillary size and reactivity. Ipsilateral constriction followed by dilatation of a pupil on the side the subdural or extradural haematoma occurs, but only in the minority. Increasingly large and sluggish pupils warn of a general increase in intracranial pressure (but rarely without increasing drowsiness and perhaps vomiting also).
- (vi) The development of these abnormalities may call for a neurosurgical opinion, as outlined above.

Group 2: Deteriorating conscious level (with or without localising neurological signs). Examination of the patient even in a coma can be surprisingly complete. Particular attention should be paid to brainstem reflexes since these may have the greater prognostic significance (p. 318). In addition to lateralised weakness, sensory loss and asymmetrical deep tendon reflexes should be looked for

Deterioration may be due either to the development of cerebral oedema or haematoma. Both may be fatal or cause secondary morbidity. Both need urgent treatment, haematomas by exploration. If the patient is deteriorating rapidly, or you do not have a CT scanner on site, you should proceed to theatre without delay. However, there is usually time to obtain a CT scan, which is really essential in these circumstances, indicating either the presence of blood, or brain swelling secondary to oedema.

The effective control of cerebral oedema should reduce secondary morbidity or mortality, and is achieved by the following means.

(i) Hyperventilation. The patient should be paralysed and ventilated to achieve a Pa_{CO_2} of 25–30 mmHg (3.3–4 kPa). This is best achieved by an initial dose of pancuronium bromide (Pavulon) of 50–100 μg/kg i.v. and followed at 1–1.5-hourly intervals by further doses of 60 μg/kg i.v. or i.m.

(ii) 20% mannitol 1.5 g/kg i.v. infused over 10 min.

(iii) Dexamethasone 0.5 mg/kg per day is still often given 6-hourly, despite the fact that it does not work![2] We do not use it.

Following the institution of these measures, arrangements should be made for continuous monitoring of intracranial pressure by, for example, a subdural catheter.

If a general anaesthetic is necessary, ketamine and halothane, both of which may raise the intracranial pressure, should be avoided. If the intracranial pressure is found to be normal, no further mannitol need be given and hyperventilation can be reduced progressively over a 24 h period. If the intracranial pressure recurs, then hyperventilation is obviously reinstituted. If the pressure remains elevated at more than 20 mmHg despite the above, barbiturate narcosis is worth trying.[9] Pentobarbitone 20 mg/kg is given as a loading dose and followed by 4 mg/kg doses to maintain the serum level between 30 μg/l and 40 μg/l (132.6 mmol/l and 176.8 mmol/l).

However, hyperventilation alone often controls the intracranial pressure adequately for 90% of the time, with occasional apparently 'spontaneous' rises to 40 mmHg or more. Some of these spontaneous rises may be triggered by the lack of sedation, increasing Pa_{CO_2}—more than 30 mmHg (4 kPa)—or hypoxaemia—Pa_{O_2} less than 85 mmHg (11.3 kPa). These causes should be looked for, and in any case a 1.5 g/kg bolus of mannitol given as above. The effect of this lasts for about 4 h. If further mannitol is necessary, a temporising measure is to give this dose as a 4 h infusion. The serum osmolality should be checked and not allowed to rise above 325 mosmol/kg. If, despite this, the intracranial pressure rises above 20 mmHg, barbiturate narcosis should be started as above.

Group 3: Initial deep coma. No eye opening, no verbal response to pain and either no motor response or abnormal flexion ('decorticate') or extension ('decerebrate') of the arms (Glasgow coma scale of 5 or less). The treatment is exclusion of an intracranial haematoma with a CT scan, and control of intracranial pressure as above, but the group here is distinguished because the prognosis is worse.

If, despite the above, the intracranial pressure remains uncontrolled, two further measures have been advocated.

(i)   Hypothermia. Whilst this may reduce the brain' metabolic demands, we are unconvinced that it has any practical beneficial effect.

(ii) Extensive craniotomy.

However, if either of these steps has to be contemplated, the patient is in a high mortality group with, in the event of survival almost inevitable major handicap. A case can be made, therefore, for withdrawal of life support at this point.

In all patients the following factors apply.

(1) The aim of management is to maintain a cerebral perfusion pressure of at least 60 mmHg. The cerebral perfusion pressure is the mean arterial pressure minus the intracranial pressure. The mean arterial pressure is, roughly: diastolic pressure + (systolic pressure − diastolic pressure)/3. If, therefore, the circulation needs support, this defines the level you should be aiming at.

(2) Fits should be treated energetically (see p. 210).

(3) Antibiotics should be given in the following circumstances.

(i)   If there is CSF or blood dripping from the ear or nose. CSF from the nose can be differentiated from mucus as only the former contains glucose (use a BM stix).

(ii) If the skull x-ray shows a fracture running into a sinus or the middle ear or the presence of intracranial air.

(iii) Where there is evidence of a basal or anterior fossa fracture (see above).

(iv)   If there are significantly (more than 5 mm) depressed fractures.

Since pneumococcus is the most likely organism to cause meningitis secondary to head trauma, penicillin 15–20 mega units/day i.v. divided into 4-hourly doses should be given until the CSF leak is stopped, the depressed fracture is elevated, or for 5 days, whichever is the longer.

(4)   The following are other complications for which you need to be alert.

(i)   Hyperpyrexia. Sponging, fanning and antipyretics including chlorpromazine are the mainstays of treatment.

(ii)   Inappropriate ADH secretion. The resulting hyponatraemia nearly always responds to fluid restriction and replacement of insensible fluid loss with normal saline.

REFERENCES

1   Butterworth J. F. *et al.* (1980). Detection of occult abdominal trauma in patients with severe head injuries. *Lancet*; **ii:** 759.
2   Fishman R. A. (1982). Steroids in the treatment of brain oedema. *N. Engl. J. Med.*; **306:** 359.
3   Grossman R. G. (1981). Treatment of patients with intracranial haematomas. *N. Engl. J. Med.*; **304:** 1540.
4   Guidelines for the initial management after head injury in adults (1984). *Br. Med. J.*; **288:** 983.
5   Hinds C. J. (1985). Prevention and treatment of brain ischaemia. *Br. Med. J.*; **291:** 7596.
6   Jeffreys R. V., Jones J. J. (1981). Avoidable factors contributing to the death of head injury patients in general hospitals. *Lancet*; **ii:** 459.
7   Jennet B., Teasdale G. (1981). *Management of Head Injuries*. Contemporary Neurology Series. F. A. Davies: Philadelphia.
8   Teasdale G., Galbraith S. *et al.* (1982). Management of traumatic intracranial haematoma. *Br. Med. J.*; **285:** 1695.
9   Ward J. O. *et al.* (1985). Failure of prophylactic barbiturate coma in the treatment of severe head injury. *J. Neurosurg.*; **62:** 383.

Syncopal attacks (faints)[1]

DIAGNOSIS

Syncope is usually defined as a transient loss of consciousness due to cerebral ischaemia, caused in turn by a reduction in blood supply to the brain.

A faint is heralded by a feeling of muzziness, objects and sounds appearing distant, and then progresses to loss of consciousness. This may be prevented if, after the warning symptoms, the sufferer lies down flat quickly enough. The patient will be strikingly pale, have a feeble, slow pulse and hypotension.

The commonest type is the so-called simple faint. This occurs, for example, in young girls at school assemblies, who have gone without breakfast, or in elderly patients who get up after a period of bed rest. It is said to be due to blood pooling in the leg veins. It is more likely to occur in people who are anaemic, hungry, tired or frightened, or who are easily affected by the sight of blood or other people fainting. Severe pain, or even the trauma of venepuncture or pleural puncture may also induce a simple faint.

(1) However, syncope may be caused by serious underlying disease.

    (i)   Any stenotic heart valve lesion.
    (ii)   Constrictive pericarditis.
    (iii) Cardiac arrhythmias (especially ventricular tachycardia and Stokes–Adams attacks).
    (iv) Myocardial infarction and pulmonary embolus.
    (v)   A severe haemorrhage.
    (vi) Involvement of the autonomic nervous system sufficient to cause a fall in arterial pressure on standing of >25 mmHg. This may be caused by drugs or an autonomic neuropathy; it is termed orthostatic syncope.
    (vii) Vertebrobasilar insufficiency (VBI). In patients with cervical spondylosis, turning of the head may cause spurs of bone to occlude the vertebral artery (but also see p. 197). The subclavian steal is a rare cause of VBI.

(2) A few more are provoked by relatively benign stimuli.

    (i)   Micturition syncope.

(ii) Cough and laugh syncope.

(iii) Carotid sinus syncope, defined as asystole of 3 s duration or more, or a fall in systolic arterial pressure of more than 50 mmHg, when the carotid sinus is stimulated.

(3) Cerebral ischaemia is one of the many triggers for a convulsion. Faints, therefore, if prolonged, can cause fits. Such patients should not be considered to have epilepsy.

(4) The following are some of the other conditions which cause transient alteration of consciousness.

(i) Transient ischaemic attacks (see p. 197).

(ii) Epilepsy (see p. 210).

(iii) Severe hypertension (see p. 44)—remember that transient losses of consciousness may be due to sudden elevation, as well as sudden drops, in arterial pressure.

(iv) Hypotension (see p. 295).

(v) Hyperventilation (see p. 335).

(vi) Cataplexy.

(vii) Paroxysmal vertigo—although in these last two consciousness is not truly lost.

MANAGEMENT

All that needs to be done in the simple faint is to lie the patient flat, or with the head slightly down, relieve any compression of the neck and maintain an airway. As indicated above, a careful history and full examination are mandatory if serious conditions are not to be missed. Investigations should include FBC, blood glucose, chest x-ray, ECG and consideration, if the attacks are repeated, of 24 h ambulatory monitoring of ECG and/or EEG.

Unfortunately, even after these worthy endeavours, a definitive diagnosis is usually possible in only about 60% of patients.[1] The encouraging thing is that in patients with no clear diagnosis, the prognosis appears excellent.

REFERENCE

1 Kapoor W. N. (1983). A prospective evaluation and follow up of patients with syncope. *N. Engl. J. Med.*; **309:** 197.

Fits

The common grand mal convulsion is usually self-limiting. All that is required is to see that the patient has an airway (turn the patient on his side and remove false teeth), does not bang against furniture or roll into the fire. The patient should not be actively restrained; well-meaning attempts to separate the teeth are unnecessary, frequently traumatic and not advised.

Repeated tonic clonic seizures without recovery between attacks or one seizure lasting more than 10 min—status epilepticus— constitute an emergency because irreversible brain damage may occur. This occurs on the basis of hypoxia, hyperpyrexia, and hypotension as well as continuing electrical activity, which itself may cause neuronal damage. In this context, it is salutary to remember that after about 20 min of continuous seizures, the metabolic demands of the brain exceed the delivery of substrate.

MANAGEMENT

General

As your patient is unconscious, you should institute the general measures necessary for the care of the unconscious patient (see p. 323).

Specific

(1) Suppressing the fits is the first priority.

  (i) The drug of choice is one of the benzodiazepines.[1] Give either clonazepam 1–2 mg i.v. or diazepam 10 mg i.v. Repeat the dose if seizure activity has not ceased within 5 min. Since diazepam precipitates when diluted, slow infusions should not be used. The same strictures probably apply to clonazepam.

  Benzodiazepines can produce respiratory depression particularly if your patient has had a recent dose of another anticonvulsant drug.

  (ii) If the benzodiazepines fail to control the fits, phenytoin sodium should be used. Infuse 15–20 mg/kg of ready-made infusion fluid over 45 min. This infusion will produce a phenytoin level of >10 μg for 24 h. This drug has the advantage of not impairing the conscious level and thus allowing an early neurological assessment. Phenytoin sodium must not be added to any other i.v. infusion as an acid precipitate may form. In the unlikely event that seizures are not controlled by the above measures, there are the following alternatives.

(iii) Chlormethiazole.[2] Use 500 ml of an 0.8% solution over 6–8 h. This drug may also cause hypotension and respiratory depression; you should neither need nor use more than 1500 ml of the 0.8% solution. Giving more is potentially dangerous as the side-effects are dose related. In the rare eventuality of having to continue with chlormethiazole, you must closely monitor blood levels.

(iv) Amylobarbitone 3–5 mg/kg i.v. at a rate not greater than 100 mg/min. This drug may rarely cause laryngospasm, depresses the conscious level and also depresses respiration. Amylobarbitone should only be used when facilities for assisted ventilation are readily available.

(v) Intramuscular paraldehyde 5 ml into each buttock is still an occasional useful standby, particularly if i.v. drugs cannot be used. Since it is painful, its use should be avoided unless the patient is unconscious. It is generally given using glass syringes since it is said to dissolve plastic. In practice it is safe to use modern plastic syringes provided the drug is given immediately. For practical purposes it does not cause respiratory depression.

If all else fails, paralyse and ventilate the patient. This will allow you to gain control of the situation. It should not be forgotten that the abnormal brain activity, which may still be continuing, may itself be a cause of neuronal damage. Attempts to control this, probably with a combination of phenytoin and chlormethiazole, should continue under continual EEG surveillance.

2) Determining the cause.

(i) In patients with epilepsy, status may be caused by either a deficiency or, rarely, an excess of their anticonvulsants. Always carry out urgent anticonvulsant estimations to determine the patient's blood levels.

    (ii)   If status is the first manifestation of seizures, a tumour is often present, and a CT scan should be performed.

    (iii)   Hypoglycaemia, hypocalcaemia, hyponatraemia[3] and hypoxia may provoke seizures. Do a BM stix, blood glucose, plasma calcium and arterial blood gases.

(3) After the fits have been controlled.

    (i)   Examine the patient, including his mouth, carefully, as injuries during the fits are common.

    (ii)   Then allow the sleep which occurs after fits to continue.

    (iii)   Initiate maintenance therapy with one of the major anticonvulsants—phenobarbitone, carbamazepine or phenytoin. Phenytoin i.v. may be given as a loading dose as above. (Never give it by i.m. injection as it is absorbed erratically.)

REFERENCES

1   Greenblatt D. J., Shader R. I. *et al.* (1983). Current status of the benzodiazepines. *N. Engl. J. Med.*; **309:** 354.

2   Harvey P. K. P., Higgenbottam T. W., Loh L. *et al.* (1975) Chlormethiazole in treatment of status epilepticus. *Br. Med. J* **2:** 603.

3   Worthley L. I. G., Thomas P. D. (1986). Treatment of hyponatraemic seizures with intravenous 29.2% saline. *Br. Med. J.*; **292:** 168.

Spinal cord compression

DIAGNOSIS

(1) This may be suggested by a history of paraparesis, sensory loss and incontinence, associated with paraesthesiae or root pain brought on or exacerbated by movement. Physical examination may establish a sensory motor, sweating or reflex level which is a guide to the level of compression.

(2) Sudden cord lesion in the absence of trauma may be caused by either intramedullary or extramedullary pathology.

Whereas the attempt to distinguish the two is an interesting clinical exercise, the conclusions are frequently wrong, particularly when the onset of symptoms is acute. The distinction is made by myelography which should be performed as soon as possible (see below). Clinical points we have found useful include the following.

    (i)   Well-localised spinal tenderness as revealed by percussion suggests epidural abscess.

    (ii) Previous and remote neurological episodes, e.g. retrobulbar neuritis, suggest demyelinating disease.

    (iii) A previous and ill-advised lumbar puncture performed in a patient with deranged coagulation suggests extradural haematoma.

    (iv) Extradural tumours are most commonly metastases from elsewhere, and extraspinal primaries should always be looked for.

MANAGEMENT

Cord compression sufficient to cause symptoms and signs for more than a few hours causes irreversible cord damage.

(1) Your neurosurgical colleagues should be consulted as soon as the diagnosis is suspected, and investigations carried out in conjunction with them.

(2) The next priority is to obtain spinal x-ray films which may reveal erosion of pedicles or vertebral bodies suggesting

extradural lesions, followed by myelography. If the technique is available, this is most safely performed above the block by a C1–2 puncture, although it is usually safe to inject contrast below the site of the lesion.

Acute ascending polyneuritis (idiopathic inflammatory polyradiculoneuropathy)

DIAGNOSIS

(1) This is made from a characteristic history of onset of weakness which involves first the legs then the arms and may spread to involve the bulbar muscles, face and respiratory muscles. This often starts 5–12 days after a mild virus infection. Commonly, weakness may be preceded by paraesthesiae and mild sensory loss. Sometimes muscle tenderness is also present. Deep tendon reflexes become absent.

(2) Differentiation is from other causes of acute weakness.

    (i) Acute poliomyelitis. The paralysis, which is nearly always asymmetrical and confined within muscle groups, is generally preceded by mild meningitic symptoms by 3–4 days. In addition, sensory signs are never found in 'polio'.

    (ii) Other causes of acute polyneuritis are distinguished by examination or simple tests. These may be:

        (a) axonal (e.g. drugs and porphyria);
        (b) demyelinating (e.g. diphtheria); or
        (c) inflammatory (e.g. the vasculitides).

        Botulism also causes generalised weakness but the onset is typically bulbar, and characteristically associated with severe constipation.

    (iii) Focal cord lesions, such as cauda equina compression or a myelopathy. These will give you a clear motor, reflex or sensory level (see p. 213).
    (iv) Myasthenia (see p. 218).
    (v) Polymyositis.
    (vi) Tick paralysis is an important consideration in some countries, including the USA and Australia. The less accessible parts of the anatomy should be carefully searched since removal of the offending tick is followed by dramatic return of power.

(3) Cerebrospinal fluid usually contains a raised protein and normal cell count at some stage of the illness, but may be normal

initially. A urine vanillyl mandelic acid (VMA) test should always be performed in children because of the association with neuroblastoma. Nerve conduction velocities are significantly slowed, at least in some portions of the nerves (since this is a disease of segmental demyelination) in most cases.

MANAGEMENT

(1) There is no specific treatment. The incidence of subsequent relapse is actually greater if steroids have been used.[3] In a recent well-controlled trial, plasma exchange was shown to speed recovery, and this may prove to be an effective therapy in selected cases.[2] Otherwise management is entirely supportive artificial ventilation being indicated urgently if paralysis of intercostal muscles or the diaphragm occurs. This happens in about a quarter of all patients during the first 3 weeks of the illness.[1]

(2) The power of the respiratory muscles may be assessed clinically in the first instance by asking the patient to count in exhalation. The patient takes a maximal inspiration, and begins to count of seconds from a clock until he is forced to take another breath. Power is impaired if the patient cannot go beyond 15 s. Whilst respiration is jeopardised this test should be performed hourly. Serial measurements of vital capacity should be made at 2-hourly intervals.[4] Most authorities would now recommend elective ventilation if the vital capacity falls to 1 litre (in an adult).

(3) You should also measure the arterial blood gases, as respiratory failure may be heralded by an insidious increase in PaCO$_2$. Absolute criteria for ventilation are a PaCO$_2$ of >45 mmHg (6 kPa) or a PaO$_2$ <75 mmHg (10 kPa).

(4) Respiratory failure can occur very rapidly with little previous distress or deterioration in the counting ability or the blood gases. Equipment for endotracheal intubation should be at hand—together with a ventilator (preferably out of sight).

(5) Respiratory embarrassment may also occur if bulbar paralysis is unrecognised. Nasal secretions and saliva accumulate in the pharynx, and intubation followed by tracheostomy with a cuffed tube may be required in order to protect the airway.

(6) Autonomic disturbances, such as gastrointestinal stasis, arrhythmias, spontaneous fluctuation of the blood pressure and

pulse rate, may occur—yet another reason for the meticulous ECG monitoring required in these patients. Acute brady-arrhythmias contribute a major share of the mortality. If these, or dropped beats, occur, a transvenous cardiac pacemaker should be passed as a matter of urgency. Propranolol 40 mg b.d. (if necessary via a nasogastric tube) may control tachy-arrhythmias.

(7) Full recovery of muscular function often occurs after total paralysis. The main factor influencing survival is meticulous and full nursing care, with special attention to tracheostomy toilet, prevention of bed sores, muscle contractures, wrist and foot drop and evacuation of bowels and bladder. Loss of sphincter control is common, and regular suppositories and an in-dwelling bladder catheter may be necessary.

(8) There is a grave danger of pulmonary emboli developing in these patients. Start subcutaneous heparin as soon as possible (see p. 17).

Details of the management of the totally paralysed patient are beyond the scope of this book.

REFERENCES

1   Hewer R. L., Hilton P. J., Smith A. C. (1968). Acute polyneuritis requiring artificial ventilation *Quart. J. Med.*; **27:** 479.

2   Hughes R. A. C. (1985). Plasma exchange for Guillain–Barré syndrome. *Br. Med. J.*; **291:** 615.

3   Hughes R. A. C., Newsom-Davis J. M., Perkin G. D., Pierce J. M. (1978). Controlled trial of prednisolone in acute polyneuropathy. *Lancet*; **ii:** 750.

4   Macklem P. T. (1986). Muscular weakness and respiratory function. *N. Engl. J. Med.*; **314:** 775.

Myasthenia gravis [1,2,3]

DIAGNOSIS

(1) This is made from a history of characteristic fatigue on continued exertion. In mild cases, power is normal after a period of rest, but then declines abnormally quickly on exercise. In more severe cases weakness is constant. The weakness may be generalised or confined to particular groups of muscles, e.g. the extraocular or bulbar muscles.

   The onset of easy fatiguability is usually insidious—occurring only at the end of the day—but occasionally it is acute. Fatiguability is demonstrated by continued use of specific muscles for a short period of time. There is no sensory loss and the reflexes are nearly always preserved.

(2) The diagnosis is confirmed by the Tensilon test, which should always be performed with an assistant and with resuscitative facilities at hand. Decide which muscle groups are weakest. Choose the three most evident and also measure the forced vital capacity (FVC). Give edrophonium (Tensilon) 2 mg i.v. stat., and if there is no sweating, salivation, lachrymation, colic or muscle fasciculation during the next minute, give a further 8 mg i.v. If these unpleasant cholinergic side-effects do occur, they may be aborted by atropine 1.0 mg i.v. Reassess the three muscle groups and remeasure the FVC within the next minute.

   Frequently the response is equivocal—some muscle groups responding dramatically and others not at all. If the overall response is indecisive, repeat the test later in the day and try to gauge the general trend. If there is still genuine doubt, the effect of Tensilon on the motor response to repetitive nerve stimulation can be studied.

MANAGEMENT

(1) Start pyridostigmine (Mestinon): 60–180 mg every 6 h may be necessary, the dose being adjusted to provide maximum response without side-effects. Oral, subcutaneous and intramuscular preparations are available as necessary.

218

(2) If swallowing is affected, place a nasogastric tube for feeding and drug and food administration.

Discussion of the place for steroids and thymectomy is outside the scope of this book.

REFERENCES

1   Dau P. C., Lindstrom J. M., Lassel C. K., Denys E. G., Shev E. E., Spitler L. E. (1977). Therapy in myasthenia gravis. *N. Engl. J. Med.*; **297:** 1134.

2   Drachman D. B. (1978). Myasthenia gravis. *N. Engl. J. Med.*; **298:** 136, 186.

3   Scadding G. K., Harvard G. W. H. (1981). Pathogenesis and treatment of myasthenia gravis. *Br. Med. J.*; **2:** 1008.

Myasthenic crisis (too little treatment)

DIAGNOSIS

(1) The myasthenic crisis is an exacerbation of weakness which most often occurs in an already diagnosed myasthenic patient. It is less frequent than formerly, now that treatment regimes are based on immunosuppression rather than anticholinesterases.

(2) However, it may occur in a previously undiagnosed patient, being precipitated by stress, emotion, infection or trauma, or by drugs which block neuromuscular transmission, e.g. streptomycin, gentamicin, kanamycin, and clindamycin. Anaesthetists are fully conversant with the prolonged action of suxamethonium in these patients.

MANAGEMENT

(1) Give edrophonium (Tensilon) as outlined on p. 218.

(2) An immediate improvement in muscle power indicates that the patient requires further anticholinesterase therapy, in addition to any other therapy he may already be receiving. Therefore, proceed as outlined for management of myasthenia.

(3) While pyridostigmine is taking effect it may be necessary to support respiration with a ventilator.

(4) Occasionally severe weakness requiring ventilatory support persists despite maximal therapy. In this situation plasmapheresis may be life saving.[1]

REFERENCE

1   Leader (1978). Plasmapheresis. *Br. Med. J.*; **1**: 1011.

Cholinergic crisis (too much treatment)

DIAGNOSIS

(1) This precipitated by excessive anticholinesterases. It occurs typically 0.5–2 h after the previous dose.

(2) The initial warning symptoms and signs are colic, sweating, salivation and fasciculation. These symptoms are sufficiently clear and drug related for it to be extremely rare for further progression to develop. However, deliberate overadministration may proceed via nervousness, drowsiness and confusion to ataxia, dysarthria, hypertension and bradycardia culminating in coma, which may be interrupted by convulsions, and finally death. The warning signs may be masked if atropine or atropine-like drugs are given with the anticholinesterases.

Helpful physical signs may be small pupils (less than 3 mm in diameter) and fasciculation which persists to a late stage.

(3) It is obviously crucial to distinguish this from a myasthenic crisis, which is the commonest cause of acute weakness in a myasthenic patient. If there is still doubt after the history and examination, give edrophonium (Tensilon) 10 mg i.v. with a ventilator at hand. If there is objective improvement, the weakness is due to a myasthenic crisis. If there is no response or a deterioration, the diagnosis is a cholinergic crisis.

MANAGEMENT

(1) Stop pyridostigmine.

(2) Give atropine sulphate 1 mg i.v. ½-hourly to a maximum of 8 mg.

(3) Maintain respiration. If acute respiratory failure occurs, the patient is ventilated in the usual way. If acute respiratory failure has not occurred, the power of the respiratory muscles may be assessed clinically by having the patient count in exhalation and perform other simple respiratory function tests (see p. 216). This should be done hourly. In addition, the blood gases should be measured regularly (the Pa_{CO_2} should be checked at least 6-hourly) and immediately if any deterioration of the counting test occurs.

221

(4) Reformation of cholinesterase should be assessed by response to the edrophonium test, which should be performed 2-hourly until a positive response of increase in muscle power occurs. At this point a small dose of oral pyridostigmine (e.g. 30 mg) should be tried.

Generalised tetanus[2,4]

DIAGNOSIS

(1) The typical case is entirely characteristic and quite unforgettable. The history is of dysphagia and stiffness and pain in the muscles of the neck, back and abdominal wall. Examination reveals hypertonia, usually greater in the extended legs than in the arms, together with painless trismus. In all but the milder cases the rigid posture is interrupted by paroxysms in which extension of the back, neck and legs and flexion of the shoulders and elbows are accompanied by the characteristic grimaces. These last up to 20 s and are painful. Rigidity persists between paroxysms, thus distinguishing tetanus from strychnine poisoning and rabies.

If the time between the onset of rigidity and the onset of spasm is no more than a few hours, subsequent paroxysms are likely to be frequent and to occur for several days.

(2) The attack may be modified by previous immunisation, the spasm remaining localised to the site of infection.

(3) The site of entry should be sought. Apart from obvious puncture wounds and infected umbilical stumps, this includes ruptured tympanic membranes, usually associated with an ear discharge.

Before treatment is instituted, the patient should be watched for a period of 10–15 min while he or she is lying relaxed in a quiet and darkened room. This, combined with your other observations, will enable you to categorise your patient—this in its turn gives you a general guideline as to how intensive your treatment will need to be. The categories are outlined below.

Grade 1. Mild spasticity, but no dyspnoea or respiratory difficulty. Sedation will probably suffice in this group.

Grade 2. More pronounced spasticity, with some impairment of breathing or swallowing, but with no generalised spasms. Here, tracheostomy as well as sedation may be needed.

Grade 3. Any patient with generalised spasms will require curarisation and artificial ventilation. In Britain, most cases fall into this category.

Your initial observations will also provide a baseline upon which the effects of treatment may be assessed.

MANAGEMENT

(1) Suppress the organism and its toxin.

    (i) Give human tetanus immunoglobulin (Humotet 100 i.u./kg i.m.—**never** i.v.)—a previous test dose being unnecessary. In the event of unavailability of human immunoglobulin, you should still give the heterologous antitetanus serum (ATS). Give 0.2 ml as a test dose, and if there is no reaction within ½ h, give 5000 units of ATS i.m. Intrathecal human tetanus immunoglobulin has been shown to be of benefit if given in early tetanus. The dose is 250 i.u. instilled intrathecally.[3]

    (ii) Give antibiotics. Metronidazole 500 mg orally, or 1.0 g rectally 8-hourly, has recently been shown to be more effective than the traditional benzylpenicillin 1 mega unit 6-hourly.[1]

    (iii) Excise all dead tissues surrounding the wound (if any) not less than 1 h after the patient has been protected by ATS and penicillin. The wound is kept open and irrigated with hydrogen peroxide or 1 × 4000 potassium permanganate solution three times a day.

(2) Treat rigidity. If the patient is developing rigidity, alternate chlorpromazine 0.5 mg/kg and phenobarbitone 1.0 mg/kg 3-hourly. It is usually necessary to give these i.m. The aim is to achieve a state of light sleep for most of the time. If this regimen is ineffective, add diazepam 0.2 mg/kg i.v. up to 5–10 mg hourly, or meprobamate 400 mg orally every 4 h. Remember that patients with rigidity have increased fluid and caloric requirements. If these drugs in combination do not produce relaxation, curarisation and artificial ventilation (IPPR) are indicated (see below).

(3) Treat spasms. Spasms are painful and dangerous as they may cause hypoxia and crush fractures of the spine and must be controlled by curarisation and IPPR. Spasms occur in response to a stimulus. This may be a distended bladder, faecal impaction or bronchial mucus, and effective control of spasms may be secured by eliminating these stimuli rather than by increasing the dose of drugs.

Swallowing also may precipitate spasms. For this reason, if the disease is likely to be severe (short periods of onset), a nasogastric tube should be passed early rather than late. Nursing attention must be kept to an absolute minimum. The single spasm which needs to be treated urgently (for example laryngospasm) may respond to chlorpromazine 100 mg i.v.

(4) Thus, to summarise, curarisation and IPPR are indicated in the following situations.

(i)   If rigidity is uncontrolled and makes breathing difficult.

(ii) If laryngospasm occurs. *This is an absolute indication.* Laryngospasm may be precipitated by attempts to pass a nasogastric or endotracheal tube and these procedures should not be attempted in the interval between the first episode of laryngospasm and the ensuing tracheostomy.

(iii) In every patient who has generalised spasm.

Complete muscle relaxation and IPPR may necessitate transfer to a specialised unit, for the chances of a successful outcome depend largely on meticulous and intensive nursing care, which may be necessary for 6 weeks or more. To the usual hazards of this sort of treatment are added other more specific complications to which patients with tetanus are especially liable, e.g. hyperpyrexia and bacterial shock, autonomic imbalance and arrhythmias. If these autonomic disturbances occur, they are treated in the usual way, and in addition heavy sedation as well as paralysis are probably beneficial.

REFERENCES

1   Ahmadsyah I., Salim A. (1985). Treatment of tetanus: an open study to compare the efficacy of procaine penicillin and metronidazole. *Br. Med. J.*; **291:** 648.

2   Edmondson R. S., Flowers M. W. (1979). Intensive care in tetanus: management, complications and mortality in 100 cases. *Br. Med. J.*; **1:** 1401.

3   Leader (1980). Tetanus immune globulins: The intrathecal route. *Lancet*; **ii:** 464.

4   Weinstein L. (1973). Tetanus. *N. Engl. J. Med.*; **289:** 1293.

Brain death[1]

The advent of prolonged ventilation has given rise to a group of patients with brain death. The non-functioning brainstem is followed, usually within a few days, by asystole, despite continued ventilation. Thus, given certain vital prerequisites, a non-functioning brainstem can be regarded as an alternative form of death—brain death.

This is an important diagnosis for two reasons.

(1) It allows organ donation to proceed.
(2) It allows ventilation to be discontinued.

The diagnosis of brain death cannot be considered until certain conditions have been excluded.

(1) Intoxication with narcotics, hypnotics or tranquillisers. Elimination of these entails a specific enquiry and full drug screen. Since there is insufficient knowledge about the effects of therapeutic concentrations of phenobarbitone (when used as an anticonvulsant) when associated with brain injury, the assessment of brainstem function for the diagnosis of brain death should be deferred until blood levels of phenobarbitone are extremely low.
(2) Hypothermia. The core (rectal) temperature should be more than 35°C.
(3) Action of relaxants (neuromuscular blocking agents). If in doubt—for example following operation—this can be excluded by finding deep tendon reflexes, spinal withdrawal reflexes or by using a peripheral nerve stimulator.

In addition, the cause of the patient's state must be known. This means both:

(1) excluding metabolic disturbances by measurement of electrolytes (including Ca^{2+}) and urea, blood glucose and acid–base balance; and
(2) having a positive diagnosis of a disorder which can cause irreversible damage. When severe trauma or major intracerebral haemorrhage has occurred, tests for brain death may be delayed for not more than a few hours. However, when brain

226

death is suspected after severe hypoxia, cardiac arrest or cerebral or fat embolism, it is prudent to wait for 24 h before making the first assessment.

DIAGNOSIS

The diagnosis should be made by two consultants or a consultant and senior registrar with expertise in the field working either together or separately. Needless to say, neither should belong to a transplant team if organ donation is anticipated.

The tests should be carried out twice, with the interval between being adequate for the reassurance of all directly concerned. The tests are as follows.

(1) Absent verbal response, spontaneous movements and pupillary light reflex. The pupils may be either midpoint or dilated. The essential factor is that they are unreactive to light.
(2) Absent corneal reflex.
(3) Absent vestibulo-ocular reflex (see p. 317). Any wax obscuring the eardrum must first be removed. Then, slowly instill 20 ml of ice-cold water into the external auditory canal. No eye movement (or other response) should occur. If the drum is obscured by local trauma, this test can be omitted and the diagnosis of brain death can still be made if all the other conditions are fulfilled.
(4) Absent oculocephalic reflex (see p. 317).
(5) No gag or cough reflex on stimulation by catheter of the pharynx or trachea, respectively.
(6) No reaction to a noxious stimulus in the area of distribution of the cranial nerves. This stimulus may be conveniently applied by firm supraorbital pressure.
(7) No ventilatory response to hypercarbia. This is most conveniently assessed by ventilating the patient with pure O_2 for 10 min followed by 5% CO_2 in O_2 for 5 min. The patient is disconnected from the ventilator and observed for 10 min while O_2 is delivered at 6 l/min by catheter into the endotracheal tube. This procedure will ensure that the Paco$_2$ will be at least 50 mmHg (6.65 kPa) while the patient is not exposed to additional hypoxia. If the patient has previous chronic respiratory failure and may normally exist on hypoxic drive, expert advice should be sought and the test carried out with careful blood gas analysis.

A checklist of these reflexes with recorded response is a useful aide memoire and entry for the notes.

Provided all these conditions are fulfilled:

(1) other tests, such as an EEG or arteriography, are unnecessary and may only confuse distressed relatives;

(2) the decision to withdraw ventilation can be taken. The timing of this becomes increasingly irrelevant provided that all those concerned with the patient appreciate that he is already dead. In one institution it is the practice to issue a death certificate at this stage—whilst the patient is still being ventilated—in order to drive the point home. The timing must be balanced between unseemly haste and subsequent recrimination on the one hand and the needless prolongation of relatives' uncertainty and suffering on the other.

REFERENCE

1   Pallis P. (1982). ABC of brainstem death. *Br. Med. J.*; **285:** 1409. (A series of articles, the first is in the *Br. Med. J.* as given here.)

Sickle cell anaemia

Sickle cell anaemia [1]

Sickle cell crisis does not occur in AS genotypes; it may be found in mixed haemoglobinopathies, such as SC disease, but more commonly it occurs in the homozygous sickle cell genotype. Distribution of the disease is throughout West and Central Africa, the West Indies and North America, and the Mediterranean littoral, and your patient will probably come from one of these areas. The disease is well recognised in its indigenous areas, and indeed may account for some of the ancient African myths. [4]

The basic problem is that deoxygenated haemoglobin tends to form gel precipitates in the red cell, causing them to sickle. Sickling is not necessarily irreversible, but the sickle cell is more sensitive to haemolysis, has a short life and, by increasing the viscosity of the blood, decreases flow in capillaries and small arterioles. The sickled cell also has a decreased O_2-carrying capacity.

People suffering from sickle cell disease spend large portions of their life in a stable state, with mean haemoglobins of 9.0 g/100 ml. A crisis can be defined as a sharp turn or definite change in the course of the disease, with development of new signs and symptoms.

DIAGNOSIS

Whatever the nature of the crisis, it is usually provoked by some stress, often an infection. This may be a urinary tract infection, stress, diarrhoea and vomiting, pneumonia, or, in the tropics, malaria. Other provoking factors are exposure to cold, anaesthesia, operations and pregnancy.

Four patterns of sickle cell crisis are described.

1) Vaso-occlusive (the commonest type). Here, hyperviscosity causes sludging, stasis and infarction of the involved tissue. The symptoms are of a sudden onset of excruciating pain, often widespread but most intense in one specific area. The commonest sites are the lumbosacral spine, chest, large joints and abdomen, where an intra-abdominal surgical crisis may be simulated. Because of the pain, your patient may be in agony. There will be widespread muscle and bone tenderness, an anaemia, a mild fever, and the white cell count is often raised to

231

20 000–60 000, even in the absence of infection. There may be a mild unconjugated hyperbilirubinaemia.

(2) Haemolytic crisis. Intravascular hypoxia causes a massive haemolysis. There will be profound anaemia (Hb 3–4 g/100 ml) and other features of haemolysis such as reticulocytosis, low haptoglobin levels, and a raised indirect bilirubin.

(3) Sequestration syndrome. In this situation there is a sudden massive painful enlargement of the liver and spleen, probably on the basis of vaso-occlusive ischaemic damage to these organs. There is an acute fall in PCV, and Hb often falls to 2–3 g/100 ml. This type of crisis is restricted to children and pregnant women,[5] and presents as cardiovascular collapse.

(4) Aplastic or hypoplastic crisis. There is abrupt cessation of function of the bone marrow, possibly again mediated through local ischaemia to the marrow. As in the haemolytic crisis, there will be profound anaemia, but none of the other features of haemolysis. This type of crisis again usually occurs in children.

Patients often have features of more than one of the above groups.

There is, at present, no effective specific treatment which reverses sickling, although many remedies are being tried. The outcome of the sickle crisis largely depends on effective treatment of the underlying cause, which must be diligently sought.

MANAGEMENT

(1) Take blood for FBP, a sickling screening test, blood gases, liver function tests, electrolytes and urea. Do blood and urine cultures and, where appropriate, viral studies. Do an MSU and stool culture if there is diarrhoea. Do a chest x-ray and an ECG.

(2) The results of your history, examination and of the above tests should allow you to determine the underlying cause of the particular episode of crisis (see above). This must be treated on its merits. Even if you do not find a specific cause, it is worth giving a broad-spectrum antibiotic such as amoxycillin 250 mg 8-hourly because of the frequent association of crisis and infection. You should also keep your patient warm.

(3) Rehydration. These patients are often fluid depleted, a fact which increases blood viscosity and thus hypoperfusion. Appropriate fluid, usually a mixture of 0.9% N saline and

dextrose, should be infused under CVP control until the patient is adequately perfused. The specific fluids you infuse will depend on the problem provoking the illness, and also on the results of your initial serum electrolytes.

(4) Acidosis. Acidosis is common in crisis, probably due to poor tissue perfusion. Acidosis also exacerbates sickling—thus it seems logical to reverse any acidosis present by giving $NaHCO_3$ as part of the infusion fluid, in amounts which you can calculate from the formula on p. 302.

(5) Oxygen. Hypoxia also aggravates sickling and if the PaO_2 is less than 80 mmHg (10.6 kPa), it is reasonable to give 100% O_2 by face mask to correct this. Hyperbaric O_2 has been tried without success.

(6) Pain relief. The pain of crisis is severe and requires appropriate analgesics; opiates (pethidine 100 mg i.m., morphine 10 mg or diamorphine 5 mg i.m.) are often necessary. You should, of course, try simpler analgesics, such as aspirin and paracetamol first.

(7) Correction of anaemia. As mentioned above, 'sicklers' usually live with Hb of around 9.0 g/100 ml. Unless there is profound anaemia (Hb <6.0 g/100 ml), transfusion is unnecessary to raise the haemoglobin. However, partial exchange transfusions to replace some of the sickle cell haemoglobin with haemoglobin in the form of fresh heparinised blood have been suggested as a mode of treatment. There is no convincing evidence for its efficiency, but in desperate circumstances it is worth trying.

(8) Specific antisickling drugs as therapeutic agents. Advances in understanding of the theoretical basis of sickling have made possible several specific therapeutic approaches.[1,2,3] So far none has been proven effective. However, as many of these treatments have been advocated, we feel that a brief survey of the mechanism and agents used is warranted, if only to warn against undue optimism. Agents tried so far are:

(i) compounds that prevent sickling by inhibiting intracellular gelation (gelation inhibitors), such as urea, dichloromethane gas, dimethyladipimidate and piracetam;

(ii) compounds which inhibit sickling independently of gelation—oral zinc cyanates.

We do not think that there is presently enough evidence to justify the use of any of these compounds.

REFERENCES

1   Alavi J. B. (1984). Sickle cell anaemia—pathology and treatment. *Med. Clin. N. Am.*; **68:** 545.
2   Dean J., Schechter A. N. (1978). Sickle cell anaemia. Molecular and cellular bases of therapeutic approaches. *N. Engl. J. Med.*; **299:** 752 (part I); 804 (part II); 863 (part III).
3   Nalbandian R. M., Henry R. L., Murayama M. *et al.* (1978). Sickle cell disease. Two new strategies. *Lancet*; **ii:** 570.
4   Onwubalili J. K. (1983). Sickle-cell anaemia: an explanation for the ancient myth of reincarnation in Nigeria. *Lancet*; **ii:** 503.
5   Serjeant G. R. (1983). Sickle haemoglobin and pregnancy. *Br. Med. J.*; **2:** 628.

Section VIII

The overdose

The overdose[1,5,6,7]

(1) This usually rests on circumstantial or third party evidence and it is therefore important to interview relatives, ambulancemen, etc., and to contact the patient's family doctor as soon as possible.

(2) It must be considered in any comatose patient.

(3) The effects may include:

    (i)   impairment of consciousness;
    (ii)   respiratory and cardiovascular depression;
    (iii) dehydration;
    (iv) hypothermia;
    (v)   convulsions.

MANAGEMENT

This does not depend at the onset on the precise identification of the drugs involved. Measures, in order of priority, are as follows.

(1) Clear and maintain an airway. Remove false teeth, food, secretions, etc., and, if necessary, insert an airway.

(2) Maintain respiration. The immediate need for assisted ventilation has to be assessed clinically, but the efficiency of ventilation can only be gauged by measuring the blood gases. Retention of CO_2—PaCO_2 > 45 mmHg (6 kPa)—and hypoxia—PaO_2 < 70 mmHg (9.3 kPa)—despite O_2 being given by an MC mask, are indications for artificial ventilation. It is unusual for a patient with a minute volume of >4 litres measured with a Wright spirometer, to require ventilation. Remember that ventilatory function may fluctuate and can deteriorate suddenly. Always remember too that your patient may have inhaled stomach contents if the protective airways reflexes have been lost (see p. 96).

(3) Maintenance of arterial pressure. If adequate tissue perfusion is not maintained, put up a CVP line and infuse plasma expanders and normal saline in the usual way (see p. 343) until the

237

CVP is in the upper range of normal. If this does not restore tissue perfusion, raise the systolic arterial pressure to above 85 mmHg by administering dopamine and/or dobutamine, or, failing these, isoprenaline (see p. 300 for dosage of both these, and the section on the hypotensive patient for a more detailed account of the pathogenesis and management of shock in overdose patients).

(4) Treat arrhythmias (see p. 23).

(5) Correct hypothermia (see p. 265).

(6) Carry out the general nursing care of the unconscious patient (see p. 323).

(7) Take blood and keep urine for drug analysis.

(8) When all this has been instituted, consider measures designed to remove the substance from the body.

(i) A stomach washout seems a logical measure in an patient who has taken a potentially toxic dose of poison. However, it is unproductive if performed more than 4 after the tablets have been taken, except in poisoning due to salicylates, tricyclic antidepressants and barbiturates when it is worth doing up to 12 h after the overdose. If the patient is conscious, consent for this procedure must be obtained, and if he or she persists in withholding consent so be it. It is dangerous to perform a stomach washout on the unconscious patient without having a cuffed endotracheal tube in place. Put the patient in the head-down position and pass a well-lubricated 30–40 French gauge orogastric tube into the stomach (it is virtually impossible to pass a large-bore tube directly into the trachea). Aspirate the stomach contents and introduce 250 ml of lukewarm water. Leave 2–3 min and then reaspirate. Repeat this procedure until 2 litres have been used, or until the lavage fluid is clear. If laryngeal spasm occurs during gastric lavage, some inhalation of stomach contents has probably taken place. In this case, aspirate the remainder of the stomach contents and withdraw the tube. If serious inhalation of stomach contents occurs, institute suction, give hydrocortisone 200 mg i.v., O_2 if necessary, broad-spectrum antibiotics, including one effective against anaerobes (see p. 309), and arrange for physiotherapy. Treat wheezing as for asthma (see p. 70).

Gastric lavage should not be undertaken in any patient

who has taken petroleum distillates, for fear of aspiration with subsequent pneumonitis. In patients who have taken corrosives, lavage should only be used if there is a serious danger of systemic effects developing, as in the case of formic acid and Paraquat.

Some authorities now favour inducing emesis as an alternative to gastric lavage. Syrup of ipecacuanha, in a dose of 30 ml for adults followed by 20 ml of water, is an effective way of so doing.

Induction of vomiting is contraindicated in poisoning due to corrosives, petroleum distillates, antiemetics (!) and in anyone whose conscious level or gag reflex is impaired.

As a general rule, the above measures are all that is required in management of overdoses. However, there are a few specific occasions when something further can be done (no more than 5% of poisoning cases); these are discussed below; and in ensuing sections.

(ii)   A forced diuresis may be worth doing in cases of poisoning due to:

    (a) long-acting barbiturates, e.g. barbitone and phenobarbitone (see below);

    (b) salicylates (see below);

    (c) amphetamines and fenfluramine and phencyclidine, the excretion of which is promoted by an acid diuresis.

(iii) Orally administered absorbents may have an occasional role once the stomach has been emptied. Activated charcoal (Medicoal) in a dose of 5–10 g every 20 min, to a maximum of 50 g, may be given in tricyclic antidepressant poisoning, and following the ingestion of some other less common agents such as sustained release theophylline preparations. Alternatively, and more conveniently, give 50 g of Carbomix, a colloidal suspension of activated charcoal.[4]

(iv) Haemoperfusion, using a column containing activated charcoal or a resin, is an efficient and safe method of removing short- and long-acting barbiturates, glutethimide, salicylates, and some other drugs from the body. Where available, it is the treatment of choice for severely intoxicated patients who fail to respond to supportive measures.[8] The levels at which the procedure may be considered are shown below.

(a) Phenobarbitone >100 mg/l.
(b) Barbitone >100 mg/l.
(c) Other barbiturates >50 mg/l.
(d) Ethchlorvynol >150 mg/l.
(e) Glutethimide >40 mg/l.
(f) Methaqualone >40 mg/l.
(g) Theophylline >60 mg/l.
(h) Trichlorethanol derivatives >50 mg/l.
(i) Salicylates >100 mg/l.

(vi) Haemodialysis only removes substances which are water soluble and which the kidney can likewise excrete. Effective forced diuresis is as efficient as haemodialysis, which should therefore only be used if there is renal failure, if charcoal haemoperfusion or resin is not available, or in cases of lithium, ethylene glycol or methyl alcohol poisoning. In methyl alcohol poisoning you should use haemodialysis if there is a metabolic acidosis, neurological symptoms or signs, a blood concentration of >0.5 g/l, or proven ingestion of more than 30 g of methanol (see p. 259).

(9) Naloxone.[3] This is a specific antidote for morphine and morphine-like compounds. It acts immediately (within 5 min) and its effect will be dramatic if your patient has taken an opiate or opiate derivative (including codeine, dextropropoxyphene and pentazocine). It will not do any harm if your patient turns out to have taken some other substance. Thus, if there is uncertainty as to which drug has been taken in any overdose with poor perfusion and poor respiration, naloxone (1.2–2.4 mg i.v. over 3 min) should be used both as a diagnostic and a therapeutic agent.

(10) Stress ulceration (see p. 93).[2]

Information as to the constituents of compounds and advice as to the management of their ingestion may be obtained from the following Poisons Information Centres.

Belfast: Royal Victoria Hospital
                  Tel: 0232 240503

Birmingham:	Dudley Road Hospital
	Tel: 021 554 3801
Cardiff:	Royal Infirmary
	Tel: 0222 569200
Dublin:	Jervis Street Hospital
	Tel: 0001 745588
Edinburgh:	Royal Infirmary
	Tel: 031 229 2477
Leeds:	General Hospital
	Tel: 0532 430715
London:	Guy's Hospital
	Tel: 01 407 7600
Newcastle:	Royal Victoria Infirmary
	Tel: 0632 325131

All these measures, complicated as they are, only constitute first aid and are relatively simple compared to dealing with the patient's problems on regaining consciousness.

REFERENCES

1   Henry J., Volans G. (1984). *ABC of Poisoning*. (A series of articles from the *Br. Med. J.* published in book form.)
2   Ivarsson L. E. (1984). Antacids and H2 receptors in the prophylaxis and treatment of erosive gastritis: clinical aspects. *Scand. J. Gastroenterol.*; **105** (Suppl.): 86.
3   Leader (1975). Naloxone. *Lancet*; **i:** 734.
4   Levy G. (1982). Gastrointestinal clearance of drugs with activated charcoal. *N. Engl. J. Med.*; **307:** 676.
5   Mathew H. (1971). Acute poisoning: some myths and misconceptions. *Br. Med. J.*; **1:** 519.
6   Prescott L. (1983). New approaches in managing drug overdosage and poisoning. *Br. Med. J.*; **287:** 274.
7   Vale J. A., Meredith T. J. (1985). *A Concise Guide to the Management of Poisoning*. London: Churchill Livingstone.
8   Vale J. A., Rees A. J., Widdop B., Goulding R. (1975). The use of charcoal haemoperfusion in the management of severely poisoned patients. *Br. Med. J.*; **1:** 5.

Salicylates [2]

The fatal dose in adults is 25 g, but death can occur from the ingestion of lesser doses. One aspirin tablet (BP) contains 300 mg of acetyl salicylic acid.

DIAGNOSIS

The patient is confused, restless, flushed, sweating, hyperventilating and complains of tinnitus. Coma is unusual unless a really massive and probably fatal overdose has been absorbed. The following metabolic changes may be present.

(1) A hypokalaemic alkalosis caused by vomiting.
(2) A respiratory alkalosis (low $Pa\text{CO}_2$, high bicarbonate) caused by hyperventilation.
(3) A metabolic acidosis, possibly caused by absorption of acid dehydration and disturbed carbohydrate, lipid and protein metabolism.
(4) Dehydration, caused by hyperventilation, sweating, vomiting reduced fluid intake, and an osmotic diuresis.
(5) Hypo- or hyperglycaemia.
(6) Pulmonary oedema, a hypersensitivity phenomenon which thus gives rise to the shock lung syndrome (see p. 91).

In young children (under 12 years of age) the acidosis is likely to predominate; adults are nearly always alkalotic when first seen. The clinical state is due to a combination of the direct effect of salicylates dehydration and altered acid–base status.

MANAGEMENT

Salicylate poisoning is one of the few overdose conditions in which early measurement of blood levels is very useful. Some patients with high blood levels show little clinical evidence of it and yet are in great danger. Symptoms occur at about 1.9 mmol (300 mg)/l. Intoxication is reckoned as severe if the level is more than 3.1 mmol (500 mg)/l and a forced alkaline diuresis may then be indicated.

Charcoal haemoperfusion or, failing that, haemodialysis may be indicated if the level is more than 6.2 mmol (1000 mg)/l, or if more than 4.3 mmol (700 mg)/l and the level is rising rapidly, or if the patient is in coma, or if there is impairment of renal function.

One value does not necessarily act as a guide to management. Far more useful are levels taken at regular intervals, e.g. every 6 h. Finally, do not rely on blood levels alone. The most important guide to the severity of the poisoning is the patient's condition. If it is bad and deteriorating, then energetic measures should be instituted whatever the salicylate level.

(1) Take blood for serum salicylate, haemoglobin and PCV, electrolytes and urea, arterial pH and PaCO$_2$. Of these results, the arterial pH is needed first. Urine should be tested for the presence of salicylates. Salicylates act as a reducing substance in Benedict's test, even after the urine has been boiled (see p. 151). A simple 'side ward' test has been described for the estimation of plasma salicylate levels.[1]

(2) A forced alkaline diuresis should be started if:

   (i)   the clinical condition is poor, i.e. the signs above are marked;
   (ii) the salicylate level is more than 1.9 mmol (300 mg)/l in children and more than 4.6 mmol (750 mg)/l in adults, or 3.1 mmol (500 mg)/l in the presence of a metabolic acidosis;
   (iii) there is a history of ingestion of more than 50 tablets.

3) Alkalinisation is unnecessary if the urine pH is already more than 8 and is dangerous if the arterial pH is more than 7.5. In either of these situations, merely start a forced diuresis (see below). If the urine pH remains acid in the face of an apparent arterial alkalosis, there is usually intracellular potassium depletion. Until this is corrected by potassium supplements, it is difficult to achieve production of an alkaline urine.

4) If the indications for forced diuresis are absent, simply observe the patient closely and encourage oral fluids.

5) If pulmonary oedema occurs, manage as for shock lung (see p. 91).

FORCED DIURESIS—ALKALINE AND ACID

1) Catheterise the bladder and keep the urine.

(2) Set up a CVP line (see p. 341) and when it reads within th
normal range (you may have to give i.v. saline and dextrose t
achieve this), assess the rate of urine flow.

(3) If the rate of urine flow is above 4 ml/min with the patien
adequately perfused, you may start the forced diuresis; if th
urine flow is less than this, give frusemide 20 mg i.v. If th
frusemide produces a urine flow of greater than 4 ml/min, it
safe to start the diuresis. If after the frusemide the urine flow
less than 4 ml/min, it is likely that renal insufficiency is presen
and the diuresis should not be undertaken. If you consider
safe to carry out the diuresis, proceed in rotation with th
following infusion.

1.26% NaHCO$_3$	— 500 ml (90 mmol NaHCO$_3$)
5% dextrose	— 500 ml
5% dextrose	— 500 ml
0.9% N saline	— 500 ml

Do not give the bicarbonate until the arterial pH is known. Give
litre of this regimen each hour for 6 h, and 500 ml/h thereafte
Provided the patient was adequately perfused prior to starting t
diuresis (which, as pointed out in (2) above, may require an init
infusion of up to 5 litres of N saline and 5% dextrose), urine outp
should approximate fluid input. If this is not the case, give i
frusemide, 20 mg as needed to keep up the urine output. If, aft
frusemide, the urinary output does not increase, or if the patie
develops fluid overload, it is probable that a degree of renal impa
ment is present (but check that the urinary catheter is not blocked
The diuresis should therefore be stopped, and charcoal haemope
fusion or haemodialysis considered. For a forced diuresis, rather th
a forced alkaline diuresis, merely substitute 0.45 N saline for
1.2% NaHCO$_3$ and proceed as above. To induce an acid diuresis, y
should give 10 g of arginine or lysine hydrochloride i.v. over 30 m
and then give oral ammonium chloride 4 g 2-hourly as necessary
keep the urine pH between 5.5 and 6.5.

(4) Give K$^+$ 26 mmol with each litre of fluid to start with.

(5) Measure and chart the following.

(i) The total fluid input and the fluid output with
cumulative total every hour.

(ii) The CVP every 30 min.

(iii) The urine pH hourly (if possible on a pH meter, which
more accurate than the universal indicator stri

Remember, the achievement of an alkaline urine is as important as the high urine output, and you must act on the regular pH readings.

(iv) The urinary and blood electrolytes and urea, and the arterial pH and PaCO$_2$ every 4 h.

(v) The serum salicylate every 6 h whilst the patient's condition is critical.

(6) Intensive monitoring is necessary because salicylate intoxication is one of the most complex metabolic states you will have to treat, and because a necessary forced diuresis, if not carefully watched, can be extremely dangerous. It follows, therefore, that the patient should be transferred to a centre where this is possible.

These measurements will allow for the following adjustments.

(i) Fluid (see above).

(ii) As soon as the urine pH is above 8, substitute 0.45 N saline for the bicarbonate.

(iii) If hyponatraemia develops, substitute N saline for one of the bottles of 5% dextrose.

(iv) Replace the measured potassium loss in the urine over 4 h, at the end of which time remeasure and repeat the process.

(7) Continue this regime, repeating the serum salicylate level, urinary and serum electrolytes and urea every 6 h. Similarly, the arterial pH and PaCO$_2$ should be measured 6-hourly until the serum salicylate level is less than 3.1 mmol/l (50 mg%).

(8) If the diuresis continues for more than 6 h, give 10 ml of 10% calcium gluconate 6-hourly. This will protect your patient against hypocalcaemic tetany, an occasional complication of prolonged alkaline diuresis.

REFERENCES

1 Brown S. S., Smith A. C. (1968). Salicylate estimation in the side room. *Br. Med. J.*; **4**: 327.

2 Proudfoot A. T. (1983). Toxicity of salicylates. *Am. J. Med.*; **75** (Suppl.): 99.

Barbiturates

DIAGNOSIS

Barbiturate overdose leads to an impaired level of consciousness, hypoventilation, hypotension, hypothermia and peripheral dilatation. As patients are often deeply comatose on admission, other causes of coma must be considered (see p. 314). A simple method for assessing blood barbiturate levels should be available to you through your biochemical laboratory.

MANAGEMENT

(1) Very few patients with barbiturate poisoning need more than supportive management. The mortality in those seriously affected is often due to irreversible changes, e.g. cerebral anoxic damage, sustained before starting treatment. It can also be due to overenergetic treatment.

(2) Charcoal haemoperfusion is probably the treatment of choice for all severe barbiturate overdoses (see p. 239).

(3) If charcoal haemoperfusion is not available, forced alkaline diuresis (see p. 244) is only indicated for substantial overdoses of phenobarbitone and barbitone. For all other barbiturates, it is of no avail.

(4) The decision to undertake charcoal haemoperfusion or a forced diuresis is primarily a clinical one. The indications are as follows.

    (i)   A history of considerable ingestion coupled with a rapidly deteriorating patient.

    (ii)   A patient who is sufficiently unconscious that there is no response to pain (as produced by rubbing the knuckle over the patient's sternum).

        The pupillary and tendon reflexes are very variable and frequently lead one to suppose that the patient is more severely poisoned than is the case.

        Inadequacy of the patient's spontaneous respiratory efforts and hypotension occurring in the absence of hypovolaemia are sinister signs.

    (iii)   If the patient's clinical state deteriorates markedly in the face of rising or constant blood barbiturate levels (see below).

Provided that reliable laboratory techniques are available, the blood barbiturate level must be assessed, as a high level may act as a warning of the seriousness of the situation, i.e. over 0.21 mmol (5 mg)/100 ml for short- and medium-acting barbiturates and 0.43 mmol (10 mg)/100 ml for phenobarbitone.

  (5) There is no place for the use of bemegride, at one time thought to be a specific barbiturate antagonist. In fact, its use has been associated with increased mortality.

Digoxin[1,2]

Acute overdosage due to this widely prescribed drug is rare, but toxicity may readily arise from its therapeutic use. The maximal therapeutic dose is about 60% of the minimal toxic dose and toxicity is especially likely to occur:

(1) if diuretics are given without potassium supplements;
(2) after a bout of diarrhoea or vomiting (both of which may cause K^+ depletion);
(3) if the patient is old and/or small;
(4) if the patient has renal failure;
(5) if other drugs, e.g. verapamil, quinidine, nifedipine or amiodarone, are being given.
(6) in a patient with coexisting hypothyroidism.

DIAGNOSIS

The patient may complain of the following.

(1) Vomiting and diarrhoea (which may exacerbate pre-existing hypokalaemia).
(2) Central nervous system problems, which may range from restlessness to frank delirium. Visual disturbances (blurring, flashes and, more specifically, problems with colour vision) occur early. Indeed, bedside testing of colour vision may be helpful in the diagnosis of toxicity.
(3) Cardiac arrhythmias, the commonest being atrioventricular block, supraventricular tachycardia, ventricular ectopics and ventricular tachycardia. Worsening heart failure may also occur.
(4) Clinically, digoxin toxicity may be difficult to distinguish from the underlying heart disorder for which it was prescribed (see 26). Blood levels may be helpful, provided the blood sample taken 6 h after the last oral dose, the normal therapeutic range being 1.0–2.0 ng/ml, with a level of above 3 ng/ml generally associated with toxic symptoms and signs. Toxicity may, however, occur at a lower level, particularly in patients above 60 years, with serum creatinine >150 μmol/l, and K <5.0 mmol/l.

MANAGEMENT

(1) In all cases of toxicity, the drug should be stopped.

(2) If the patient is nauseated and is having occasional ventricular ectopics, it is usually sufficient to discontinue the drug for a day or two. The effect of digoxin can be partially reversed by potassium, and 20–40 mmol of KCl per day orally should be given.

(3) If the situation is more urgent (e.g. the patient has persistent vomiting, is in heart failure, heart block or has an arrhythmia compromising output), the following two measures should be instituted.

   (i) Intravenous K^+ should be given: 40 mmol K^+ in 5% dextrose should be infused over 1 h, with continuous ECG monitoring. The drip should be stopped immediately if sinus rhythm returns or if peaking of T waves (evidence of hyperkalaemia) occurs. Up to 120 mmol K^+ may have to be given. If the initial serum K^+ was normal, it is wise to infuse the K^+ in a 500 ml solution of 20% dextrose with 30 units of soluble insulin added.

   (ii) Magnesium also counteracts the toxic effects of digoxin on the myocardium. Therefore, as well as giving K^+, give 2 ml of 50% $MgSO_4$ diluted to 50 ml over the course of 1 h, and repeat as necessary.

(4) If the above therapy is unsuccessful, further treatment will be required. Propranolol 1–2 mg i.v. slowly is said to be the drug of choice for digoxin-induced ectopics and tachycardias. Phenytoin 3.5–5.0 mg/kg by slow i.v. injection to a maximum of 50 mg in 1 min is an alternative.

   Atropine 0.6 mg i.v. may counteract digoxin-induced bradycardias. Transvenous pacing may be required for persistent heart block, or a widening PR interval despite K^+ therapy.

(5) In patients with digoxin-induced arrhythmias, DC cardioversion may provoke either heart block or, rarely, resistant ventricular tachycardia. So cardioversion should not be used lightly in such patients. However, in the face of a life-threatening arrhythmia, DC reversion (see p. 26) should be undertaken. Very low energies, e.g. 10 J, should be used to start with. Since heart block may occur, transvenous pacing should be readily available.

(6) Digoxin undergoes an enterohepatic circulation, and cholestyramine can bind it in the gut. This provides a possible, but as yet untested, way of getting rid of digoxin.

(7) Incomplete (Fab fragment) antidigoxin antibodies have the advantage of nullifying the effect of digoxin without being immunogenic. Now commercially available, they may ultimately provide the most satisfactory answer to this problem

REFERENCES

1   Aronson J. K. (1983). Digitalis intoxication. *Clin. Sci.*; **64:** 253

2   George C. F. (1983). Digitalis intoxication. *Br. Med. J.*; **286:** 1533.

Iron[1]

Some iron tablets look like certain well-known sweets, and sometimes small children unwittingly take handfuls of them. A dose of 3 g as elemental iron may be fatal (a 200 mg tablet of ferrous sulphate contains 60 mg and a 300 mg tablet of ferrous gluconate contains 36 mg of elemental iron). The features of iron poisoning are as follows.

DIAGNOSIS

(1) Acute haemorrhagic gastroenteritis up to 3 h after ingestion and then often after an interval of apparent spontaneous recovery.
(2) Acute encephalopathy (up to 24 h).
(3) Occasionally acute hepatic necrosis (up to 3 days).
(4) Following recovery from these reactions there may be subsequent cicatricial strictures of the gut.

MANAGEMENT

If treatment is started as soon as possible, the complications of (2) and (3) above may be avoided.

(1) Give desferrioxamine 2 g i.m.
(2) Wash out the stomach and leave behind desferrioxamine 5–10 g in 50 ml of fluid.
(3) Take blood for haemoglobin and PCV electrolytes, and urea and serum iron.
(4) If a history of ingestion of considerable quantities is obtained or vomiting or bloody diarrhoea occurs, or serum iron is above 90 μmol/l (500 μg%), give desferrioxamine 15 mg/kg per h i.v. to a maximum of 80 mg/kg per 24 h. This, if necessary, may be infused added to blood.
(5) Continue giving desferrioxamine 2 g i.m. 12-hourly until the serum iron is less than 90 μmol/l (500 μg%) and the clinical state is satisfactory. This will have to be continued for 24 h as

iron which is initially taken up by the reticuloendothelial system is released 12 h later.

(6) Blood may need to be given if haemorrhage has been severe. If diarrhoea has been severe, 0.9% saline, 5% dextrose and potassium supplements may need to be given.

REFERENCE

1 Lavender S., Bell J. A. (1970). Iron intoxication in an adult. *Br. Med. J.*; **2:** 406.

Tricyclic and tetracyclic antidepressants[3]

Today, drugs of this group are amongst those most commonly taken in overdose.

DIAGNOSIS

Clinical features include depression of consciousness, which is seldom severe, dilated and sometimes unequal pupils responding poorly to light, increased muscle tone which may be accompanied by tremor or frank convulsions, pronounced tendon reflexes and urinary retention. Additionally, cardiac dysrhythmia and respiratory depression are important features of overdose with this group of drugs.

MANAGEMENT

(1) This is essentially supportive care (as outlined on p. 237) as there is no known way of accelerating the elimination of these drugs.

(2) Prompt and adequate correction of any acidosis by giving appropriate doses of bicarbonate intravenously.[2]

(3) Monitor ECG. Prolonged inter- and intraventricular conduction times lead to the appearance of bizzare complexes on the ECG, often simulating ventricular and supraventricular tachycardia with aberrant conduction. These arrhythmias do not have the same prognostic significance as those following myocardial infarction or in ischaemic heart disease. Since the majority of conventional antiarrhythmic agents are in fact toxic, their use should be avoided if at all possible, particularly if the cardiac output is maintained. If necessary, volume repletion and an ionotropic agent, such as dobutamine 5–40 µg/kg per litre by i.v. infusion, may be used to maintain the arterial pressure.

(4) It is likely that 10–50 g of effervescent charcoal taken orally (or by a nasogastric tube if the patient is unconscious) will adsorb

any residual drug in the gastrointestinal tract, thus minimising any absorption which might take place after you first see the patient.[1]

(5) Convulsions should be controlled without delay by conventional means (see p. 210), but hypoxia should first be excluded as the primary cause.

REFERENCES

1   Crome P. *et al.* (1983). Activated charcoal in tricyclic antidepressant poisoning: pilot controlled trial. *Clin. Toxicol.*; **2:** 205
2   Leader (1976). Sodium bicarbonate and tricyclic antidepressant poisoning. *Lancet*; **ii:** 838.
3   Meredith T. J., Vale J. A. (1985). Poisoning due to psychotropic agents. *Adverse Drug Reactions and Acute Poisoning Reviews*; **4:** 83.

Paracetamol

An overdose (e.g. 15 g or more) of this drug may give rise to no more than nausea as an initial symptom, but may later cause acute hepatic necrosis and failure. Approximate blood levels, after which hepatic necrosis is likely, are given in Fig. 22. If these blood levels are exceeded, treatment with a specific protecting agent should be considered. About 10% of patients consume sufficient paracetamol to cause liver damage. Without treatment, one in five of these would die of liver failure. In this group, the liver function tests are maximally abnormal at 3 days after the overdose; a prothrombin time of >25 s 48 h post-poisoning is prognostically ominous.

MANAGEMENT

(1) If the patient is at risk of hepatic damage, and presents within 10–12 h of the overdose, methionine may be given orally. Give 2.5 g as the initial dose, followed by three more doses, each of 2.5 g, at 4-hourly intervals.[4] If your patient is vomiting, or oral methionine is not available, use N-acetylcysteine (see below).

(2) Alternatively, N-acetylcysteine by the i.v. route at an initial dose of 150 mg/kg in 200 ml 5% dextrose over 15 min, followed over the next 4 h by a second dose of 50 mg/kg in

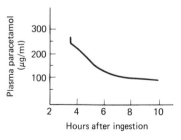

Fig. 22 Plasma paracetamol concentration after overdosage. Treatment is indicated in patients with concentrations exceeding those shown in the graph. (Reproduced with permission from L. F. Prescott *et al.* and the editors of the *Lancet*.)

0.5 litres of 5% dextrose, and finally, over 16 h, a dose of 100 mg/kg in 1 litre of 5% dextrose.[3]

(3) If more than 10 h have elapsed since ingestion, the use of a specific antidote is contraindicated, for not only is it unlikely to be effective, but it may be harmful. In these circumstances, haemoperfusion over activated charcoal may be considered, but specialist advice should be sought.

REFERENCES

1 Gillette J. M. (1981). An integrated approach to the study of the clinically active metabolites of acetaminophen. *Arch. Intern. Med.*; **141**: 375.

2 Prescott L. F. (1983). Paracetamol overdosage—pharmacological considerations and clinical management. *Drugs*; **25**: 290.

3 Prescott L. F., Illingworth R. N., Critchley J. A. J. H., Stewart M. J., Adams R. D., Proudfoot A. T. (1979). Intravenous N-acetylcysteine: the treatment of choice for paracetamol poisoning. *Lancet*; **ii**: 1097.

4 Vale J. A., Meredith T. J., Goulding R. (1981). Treatment of acetaminophen poisoning—the use of oral methionine. *Arch. Intern. Med.*; **141**: 394.

Distalgesic (coproxamol)[1,2]

This analgesic is being prescribed, and thus also being taken in overdose, with increasing frequency. All this despite the fact that there is little evidence that it is in any way superior to other simple analgesics. Each tablet contains 32.5 mg dextropropoxyphene and 325 mg paracetamol.

DIAGNOSIS

The patient presents with respiratory depression and coma; 10% may have epileptic attacks. The finding of constricted pupils on examination is highly discriminating, as unless the patient is deeply unconscious, poisonings other than with opiates are associated with dilated pupils.

MANAGEMENT

(1) Dextropropoxyphene is closely related to methadone, and thus any cardiorespiratory depressant effects are reversible with naloxone (see p. 72). Remember that the metabolites of dextropropoxyphene have long half-lives, and there is a tendency for late and unpredictable deterioration to occur. As the duration of action of naloxone is relatively short, repeated doses may be necessary.

(2) The paracetamol level should be measured, and appropriate therapy started as necessary (see p. 255).

REFERENCES

1   Proudfoot A. T. (1984). Clinical features and management of distalgesic overdose. *Hum. Toxicol.*; **3:** 853.
2   Young J. B. (1983). Dextropropoxyphene overdose. *Drugs*; **26:** 70.

Beta-blockers[1]

These may produce hypotension, bradycardia and myocardial depression leading to cardiogenic shock.

MANAGEMENT

Conventional advice is to give atropine (which does not, however, work) and isoprenaline, which may be required in massive doses of up to 50 μg/min. The cardiac stimulant action of glucagon may be helpful here, and is certainly worth trying. Give glucagon 5–10 mg i.v. by bolus injection followed by an infusion sufficient to maintain an adequate cardiac output.

Hyperglycaemia, a further effect of glucagon, does not seem to be a problem, but you should monitor the blood sugar.

REFERENCE

1   Prescott L. F. (1983). New approaches in managing drug overdosage and poisoning. *Br. Med. J.*; **287:** 276.

Methanol[1]

The patient suffering from methanol overdosage presents with confusion, ataxia, epigastric pain and vomiting and blurring of vision. A
metabolic acidosis with a large anion gap (see p. 169) and coma may
supervene.

MANAGEMENT

Traditional methods directed at correcting the acidosis (with HCO_3),
and inhibiting the oxidation of methanol to aldehydes by using ethyl
alcohol, may now be aided by the use of haemodialysis. This should
be undertaken if your patient is known to have ingested more than
30 g of methanol, or has a level of 0.5 g/l.

REFERENCE

1   Leader (1983). Methanol poisoning. *Lancet*; **i:** 910.

Organophosphate poisoning

The organophosphates are commonly used as insecticides, particularly in developing countries. Overdose, either intentional or accidental, is common.

These compounds irreversibly bind to the cholinesterases in the body. The cholinesterases normally inactivate acetylcholine, so when they are not working, acetylcholine levels rise; the effect of organophosphate intoxication is due to an increase in the levels of acetylcholine.

Exposure to these organophosphate compounds is through the skin, by inhalation (usually accidental in farm workers) or ingestion (usually intentional). They vary in toxicity, malathion being of low toxicity, parathion being of high toxicity.

DIAGNOSIS

(1) The overactivity of acetylcholine, most pronounced at autonomic post-ganglionic fibres, gives rise to the following symptoms.

    (i)   Bradycardia and hypotension.
    (ii)   Miosis.
    (iii) Vomiting, abdominal colic and diarrhoea.
    (iv) Dyspnoea due to airways obstruction and respiratory muscle dysfunction.
    (v)   Bronchial hypersecretion, excessive salivation and sweating.
    (vi) Fasciculation and convulsions.
    (vii) Disorientation, progressing to coma and death.

(2) The setting and clinical findings are usually sufficient to make the diagnosis. However, this can be confirmed by measuring the blood pseudocholinesterase level which is reduced, commonly to very low levels. The breath also has a characteristic odour.

(3) It is important to remember that serum pseudocholinesterase levels are neither a good marker of the severity of poisoning nor a good predictor of recovery. Red cell cholinesterase level, reflecting tissue cholinesterases, are considerably more helpful.

in this regard. Even so, these levels can be depressed to 60% of normal without clinical signs, especially if the patient has been handling organophosphates previously.

MANAGEMENT

Non-specific

(1) The most common immediate cause of death is respiratory failure. Check the vital capacity hourly, which will give you a lead on the progression of the illness, and blood gases. Respiratory failure, as defined by abnormal Pao_2 and $Paco_2$ (see p. 67), requires ventilatory support. Remember that sudden deterioration in the respiratory status is common; hence the need to measure vital capacity, peak flow and blood gases regularly.

(2) Remove contaminated clothing.

(3) Bathe your patient. Organophosphates are excreted in sweat, and may be resorbed through the skin. Some authorities recommend hourly bathing.

(4) Your patient may be hypovolaemic due to excessive fluid loss through diarrhoea, sweating and salivation. Appropriate circulatory support, monitored using a CVP line, should be given. Remember that the lungs may appear 'wet': this is not due to fluid overload, but to excessive bronchial secretions, which you hope to control with atropine (see below).

Specific

(1) Atropine is the mainstay of treatment. The questions are, how much and for how long?

    (i) *How much?* You should start with 1.2–2.0 mg i.v. stat. and then at 10 min intervals. You will almost certainly have to use this order of dose for the first 24 h; after this you may be able to reduce it. Monitoring is on the basis of the development of atropinic side-effects. None is absolutely reliable, but a dry mouth, a pulse rate above 100 beats/min, and decreasing secretions in the lungs indicate satisfactory atropinisation. When these features appear, you can reduce the dose to 0.6–1.0 mg and increase the interval between doses to 20–30 min.

(ii) *For how long?* You may need to continue atropine for up to 2 weeks. After each 6–12 h period, provided there is adequate atropinisation, further increase the dose intervals to 1 and then 2 h. You can then give atropine orally 4-hourly, and so titrate the amount downward gradually over a 2 week period.

(2) Atropine, whilst blocking the effects of acetylcholine at postganglionic nerve endings, does not affect brain cholinesterase. This has two main consequences.

(i) If your patient is seen within 12 h of the overdose, give an oxime which does have an effect on brain cholinesterase. Oximes act by deconjugating the organophosphate from the cholinesterase enzymes, a process which becomes more difficult once more than 12 h have elapsed after the overdose. Use either of the following.

(a) Obidoxime (Toxogonin) is the most potent preparation available and it crosses the blood–brain barrier. Give 3–6 mg/kg body weight i.v., repeated 4-hourly for 12–24 h, depending on the response.

(b) Pralidoxime is an acceptable alternative. Give 30–60 mg/kg body weight i.m. 4-hourly, or i.v 4-hourly (do not exceed 500 mg/min) for 12–24 h, depending on response.

(ii) Atropine does not have a predictable effect on the disorientation and confusion induced by organophosphates. As an excess of atropine may also cause confusion, you may be faced with a confused, disorientated and sometimes violent patient, and not know whether this is due to an excess of atropine. Our experience is that such symptoms occurring within the first 3 days are due to the effect of the overdose and not the treatment. Therefore, in these circumstances, be very wary before reducing atropine.

(3) Diazepam 5–10 mg i.m. or i.v. may be given for muscle cramp and twitching. It has been shown to act synergistically with pralidoxime to reduce the severity of CNS symptoms.

(4) Remember that many of the accidental overdoses are due to inadequate safety precautions. Enquire about the working environment and take appropriate steps if this is deemed dangerous.

Hypothermia

Hypothermia [2,3,4,5]

Hypothermia has been defined as a central (usually rectal) temperature of less than 35°C (95°F).

DIAGNOSIS

(1) Hypothermia can only be diagnosed using a low-reading rectal thermometer. A recording of 33°C (91.4°F) should arouse suspicion, for the true temperature may be lower as this is the lowest reading on an ordinary thermometer.

(2) Hypothermia may be the sole cause of coma in anyone exposed to a low temperature.

(3) Alternatively, it may complicate coma from other causes, especially hypoglycaemia, strokes, alcohol and chlorpromazine overdosage. It may either precipitate or be caused by myxoedema (see p. 176) and hypopituitary coma (see p. 164).

(4) Below about 31°C (88°F), shivering gives way to muscular rigidity accompanied by a slow pulse and respiration and hypotension. Acidosis, caused by hypoventilation and excessive lactic acid production, may be present. The ECG shows J (junctional) waves[1] (Fig. 23). Ventricular fibrillation can occur at any temperature below 30°C (86°F).

MANAGEMENT

(1) Take blood for full blood count, electrolytes and urea, serum amylase, blood glucose, blood gases and thyroid function. Measure the rectal temperature half-hourly. Further measures are:

    (i)   the general care of the unconscious patient (see p. 323);
    (ii) treatment of the hypothermia and its complications.

(2) Rewarming. The biblical method where the beautiful Shulamite, Abishag, was laid beside the freezing David, should seldom be used.

    If hypothermia occurs in a young patient as an acute episode,

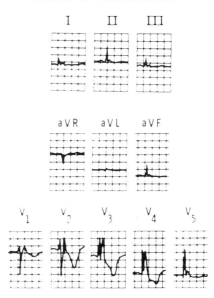

Fig. 23 The ECG in hypothermia. (Reproduced with permission from Drs D. Emslie-Smith, G. E. Sladden and G. Stirling and the publishers of the *British Heart Journal*.)

for example immersion in cold water, put the patient in a bat at 45°C (113°F) and then, when the core temperature has rise to 33°C (91°F), into a bed with warm blankets.

(3) In other circumstances, controversy over the rate of rewarmin still exists. Traditionally, slow warming (0.8°C/h) has bee advocated. This is achieved by nursing the patient, covere with blankets, in a room at 26–29°C (79–84°F). However, th morbidity from hypothermia is directly related to the tim spent hypothermic. Therefore, more rapid warming at a rate about 1.5°C/h may be advisable. The problem here is that th vasodilatation and consequent relative hypovolaemia whic occurs on rewarming will be more marked with rapid rewarm ing. However, as you should anyway nurse your patient in th ITU and monitor the cardiovascular system closely, this shou not constitute a problem for you. Therefore, we opt for fa rewarming, as this seems more logical to us. This can

achieved by a combination of electric blankets, warm-air fans, and the warming of inspired gases and i.v. fluids.

(4) In addition to rewarming your patient, correct the following factors which can complicate hypothermia.

(i) Hypotension. This may be caused by the following.

    (a) Steroid insufficiency. Take blood for a cortisol level and then give 200 mg of hydrocortisone i.v. followed by 50 mg i.v. 4-hourly if there is an initial response.

    (b) Relative circulatory insufficiency produced by peripheral vasodilatation as rewarming proceeds (see above). Insert an arterial and CVP line, and infuse plasma in the usual way (see p. 343) until the CVP is normal. In severe hypothermia—core temperature below 30°C (86°F)—a Swan–Ganz catheter to measure PCWP is useful in helping you to assess fluid replacement (see p. 346).

    Avoid using catecholamines in this condition if possible: they are especially likely to cause ventricular arrhythmias.

(ii) Hypoventilation. This may need treatment (indicated, as always, by measurement of the arterial blood gases). Hypothermia may lead to dependence on hypoxic drive (as in some patients with chronic respiratory failure), and artificial ventilation may be necessary.

(iii) Acidosis, which may be severe. Calculate the base deficit (see p. 302) and restore with the appropriate amount of sodium bicarbonate in the usual way.

(iv) Ventricular fibrillation. As the O_2 demand of tissues is reduced by about 7%/°C fall in temperature, it may be worthwhile continuing cardiac massage for longer than usual in hypothermic patients. If ordinary methods of direct current reversion do not cause a return to sinus rhythm, it has been suggested that a thoracotomy should be performed and the pericardium irrigated with warm saline—internal defibrillation then being attempted (see p. 8).

(v) Pulmonary oedema is an occasional complication of rewarming, due to leaky capillaries, and is thus really a form of 'shock lung' (see p. 91). Intermittent positive pressure ventilation may be necessary.

(vi)   Infection. A broad-spectrum antibiotic should be given
        i.v. as pneumonia usually develops.
(vii) Acute pancreatitis, the incidence of which is over-
        estimated.
(viii) Blood glucose levels. These are often abnormal in
        hypothermia; they may be either high or low, and should
        be treated accordingly.

REFERENCES

1   Emslie-Smith D., Sladden G. E., Stirling G. R. (1959). The
     significance of changes in the ECG in hypothermia. *Br. Heart
     J.*; **21:** 343.
2   Exton-Smith A. N. (1973). Accidental hypothermia. *Br. Med.
     J.*; **4:** 727.
3   Hervey G. R. (1973). Physiological changes occurring in
     hypothermia. *Proc. R. Soc. Med.*; **66:** 1053.
4   Leader (1978). Treating accidental hypothermia. *Br. Med. J.*
     2: 1383.
5   Paton B. C. (1983). Accidental hypothermia. *Pharmacol.
     Ther.*; **22:** 331.

Acute febrile illness

The acutely febrile patient

(1) Thermoregulatory neurons in the hypothalamus, sensitive to endogenous pyrogen (see below), control body temperature. In a healthy person there is a daily variation around the normal temperature of 37.0°C (98.6°F), the evening temperature being 0.5–1.0°C higher than in the morning.

(2) Endogenous pyrogen is a small molecular weight protein released by monocytes and many of the fixed phagocytic cells of the body, such as Kuppfer cells.

(3) The release of endogenous pyrogen is activated by:

    (i)   many infective agents;
    (ii)   lymphokines formed by antigenic sensitisation of lymphocytes;
    (iii)   soluble complexes.

Some tumours produce endogenous pyrogen-like proteins.

(4) The sudden onset of a fever below 40.5°C (105°F) is not of itself harmful. It only requires lowering if it:

    (i)   produces a tachycardia sufficient to cause cardiac embarrassment (usually only in patients with pre-existing cardiac disease);
    (ii)   produces febrile convulsions (usually in children);
    (iii)   makes your patient extremely uncomfortable.

So your main concern with a fever of this level is diagnostic; an approach to this problem is outlined below.

(5) A fever above 41.1°C (106°F) may, of itself, cause an encephalopathy, and therefore requires treatment. This extreme hyperpyrexia is usually caused by the following.

    (i)   Heat stroke, which is defined as a rapid rise in temperature to above 40°C (104°F) following exposure to intense heat. Your patient's skin is hot and dry, as there is generalised anhydrosis, and initial confusion may progress to coma. It is thought to be due to a control failure of the sweating mechanism.
    (ii)   Primary neurological lesion of the pons or hypothalamus involving the thermoregulatory centre.

271

    (iii)   Only rarely, by infection. Falciparum malaria is the most important of these, and should always be excluded in hyperpyrexial patients.

(6) Each 1°C rise in fever increases the pulse rate by about 10–1 beats/min and the respiratory rate by about 3–5/min.

MANAGEMENT OF FEVER

(1) If the temperature is below 40.5°C (105°F) and you deem treatment necessary (see (4) above) you should:

    (i)   commence tepid sponging, cooling with a fan and, available, use cooling blankets;

    (ii)   give aspirin 300–600 mg 4-hourly (but not to anyone under 14 years old). Alternatively, paracetamol, 500 m 4-hourly may be used.

(2) If the oral temperature is above 41.1°C (106°F), this constitute a medical emergency in its own right (see (5) above). Your aim is to reduce the oral temperature to 38.3°C (101°F) within a hour. You should take the following steps.

    (i)   Immerse your patient in a bath containing cool water an ice chips.

    (ii)   Take the temperature at 5 min intervals.

    (iii) When it has dropped to 38.3°C (101°F), nurse you patient on a bed in a cool room. The temperature usual then continues to fall to around 37°C (98.6°F).

    (iv) If, after the initial rapid cooling, the temperature starts t rise again, it can usually be controlled by the methoc outlined in (1) above.

    (v)   Where restlessness is a problem, chlorpromazir 25–50 mg i.v. can be used in addition to the physic methods of treatment.

    (vi) If, during cooling, your patient becomes shocked, yc should institute measures as outlined on p. 297.

DIAGNOSIS OF ACUTE PYREXIAL ILLNESS

(1) Worldwide, viral illnesses are the commonest cause of acu pyrexial illness. These give rise to pyrexia alone, or accom

panied by non-specific symptoms of headache, abdominal pain, vomiting, sore throat and nasal discharge. Such viral illnesses are self-limiting, usually settling within 3–4 days, and are not at present amenable to specific therapy.

(2) Fever may also be the initial symptom of other more serious infections and if associated with rigors, bacteraemia or parasitaemia is likely. The range and diversity of these vary considerably from one geographical location to another, and doctors should apprise themselves of the local circumstances. Trypanosomiasis causing sleeping sickness in central Africa and various of the haemorrhagic fevers specific to certain localities are examples of locally relevant pyrexial illnesses.

(3) Notwithstanding particular local circumstances, acute febrile illnesses of consequence (temperature >39.5°C (102°F) and often rigors) frequently have associated clinical features which allow you to make an informed decision about diagnosis and treatment.

   (i)   The clinical features may point to a specific system involved with the infection.

       (a) Headache, photophobia, stiff neck and positive Kernig's sign suggest meningitis or meningoencephalitis (see p. 328).

       (b) Pleuritic pain, cough and disproportionate dyspnoea suggest pneumonia (see p. 99).

       (c) An acutely painful joint suggests a bacterial arthritis (see p. 332)

       (d) Lower abdominal tenderness associated with an offensive vaginal discharge in a sexually active woman suggests pelvic inflammatory disease. The gonococcus (a gram-negative coccus) must be excluded, but multiple organisms, including anaerobes, may be involved. Therapy should include metronidazole, and a broad-spectrum antibiotic active against Chlamydia, and an antibiotic active against the prevailing gonococcus. Septic abortion has a similar presentation, with the addition of an enlarged tender uterus and dilated os. The likely organisms are again multiple, and include anaerobes. These patients are best treated with a penicillin, metronidazole and a broad-spectrum antibiotic such as gentamicin or chloramphenicol.

(e) A sore throat, with enlarged exudative tonsils, enlarged lymph nodes, difficulty in swallowing and prostration, suggests a bacterial tonsillitis (usually a β-haemolytic streptococcus, and therefore sensitive to penicillin). An associated erythematous rash, especially on the face and flexor surfaces of the arms and legs, which desquamates after fading, is characteristic of scarlet fever. Diphtheria is now uncommon. If difficulty in breathing is associated with a sore throat, consider acute epiglottitis. This is usually caused by the gram-negative rod *Haemophilus influenzae* and responds to chloramphenicol.

(f) Local skin sepsis, either a cellulitis (most commonly due to a β-haemolytic streptococcus) or a boil (most commonly due to *Staphylococcus aureus*), may progress to septicaemia. Penicillin will be active against the streptococcus, but the staphylococcus may be penicillinase-producing, and, if you suspect this, you should use flucloxacillin as well.

(g) Acute tenderness over a bone, with associated local swelling, suggests osteomyelitis, the treatment of which is initial drainage and flucloxacillin, on the assumption that the causal organism is *Staphylococcus aureus* and may produce penicillinase.

(h) Bloody diarrhoea associated with a high fever is often infective, and implies not only local invasion of the colon, but also bloodstream invasion by the organism. In these circumstances, a broad-spectrum antibiotic active against the likely pathogens—the shigellas (ampicillin 50 mg/kg per day in four divided doses), campylobacter (erythromycin 500 mg q.d.s.) and, less commonly, the non-typhoid salmonella (ampicillin as above)—should be started. Chloramphenicol 1 g 6-hourly orally or i.v. is effective against all the above. *Entamoeba histolytica* should first be excluded by examining a fresh stool—if present, metronidazole 400 mg t.d.s should be started.

(i) Pain in the loin, frequency and dysuria suggest urinary tract infection. If this is community acquired, the infecting organism is likely to be an *Escherichia coli* (a gram-negative rod) sensitive to sulphonamide (such as sulphamethizole 200 mg five times each day) or ampicillin 500 mg q.d.s.

(j) A painful enlarged liver, usually without jaundice but with signs at the base of the right chest, suggests a liver abscess which may be amoebic. Amoebic abscesses respond well to metronidazole 800 mg t.d.s., and aspiration is now considered to be unnecessary. There is not always a history of preceding diarrhoea. In 50% of bacterial liver abscesses there is no obvious primary site; there are usually a number of different bacteria involved, some of which are anaerobes. Bacterial abscesses should be aspirated, and metronidazole and ampicillin given pending the results of culture.

(k) Jaundice. Apart from yellow fever, viral hepatitis is unlikely to cause significant pyrexia. Malaria, leptospirosis and Q fever are specific infections which are commonly associated with jaundice. Septicaemias may also cause a non-specific toxic hepatitis.

(l) Abdominal pain. The acute infective diarrhoeas often cause pain, as may cholecystitis and diverticulitis, where there will also be localised tenderness and often a mass.

(m) Earache, a red drum or a discharging ear, suggests an acute otitis media, usually caused in adults by the gram-positive diplococcus *Streptococcus pneumoniae*, and therefore responsive to penicillin.

(n) A herpes simplex eruption is commonly associated with malaria, bacterial meningitis, pneumococcal pneumonia, leptospirosis and severe viral infections. It is uncommon in other acute febrile illnesses.

(ii) In addition, the clinical features may suggest a possible cause through association.

(a) Contact with animals, either recreational, occupational or inadvertent, should be asked for.

Anthrax, caused by *Bacillus anthracis*, a gram-positive rod, is common amongst the cattle-rearing peoples of East and Central Africa, and in those intimately involved in the handling of hides. There may be a characteristic malignant pustule and surrounding oedema, but the respiratory variety occurs without the pustule. Penicillin 4 mega units 6-hourly is the treatment of choice.

Brucellosis, a septicaemic illness caused by a gram-negative rod conveyed to humans through intimate contact with infected goats and cows, or through consuming infected milk or cheese, responds to tetracycline or chloramphenicol. A leucopenia is characteristic.

Leptospirosis. The leptospira, finely coiled motile spirochaetes, are concentrated in the urine of rodents. Humans, when in contact with infected non-salt water, are at danger, and so the disease particularly affects sewer workers, farmers, and those in abattoirs. Penicillin 4–10 million units a day may be helpful.

Psittacosis, caused by the obligate intracellular organism *Chlamydia psittaci*, and usually transmitted to humans by the otherwise inoffensive parrot family, gives rise to an atypical pneumonia responsive to tetracycline 500 mg q.d.s.

Q fever is an illness caused by the rickettsial organism *Coxiella burneti.* Humans are infected by inhalation or ingestion of the organism after exposure to infected goats, cattle or sheep. Farmers and those involved in animal husbandry are at risk. Unpasteurised milk, though often contaminated with *Coxiella burneti*, does not seem to transmit the disease. Q fever responds to tetracycline 500 mg q.d.s.

(b) If there is evidence that your patient is from an overcrowded, unhygienic, deprived community, particularly one recently overtaken by any social calamity, you should think of the following pyrexial illnesses.

Plague. Yersinia pestis is the gram-negative bacillus causing plague. Here the disease is transmitted to humans when there is close cohabitation between infected fleas, rats, humans and their domestic animals. The septicaemic illness is associated with swollen, tender and sometimes discharging local lymph node (the bubo). The disease responds briskly to tetracycline 500 mg q.d.s. and streptomycin.

Epidemic louse-borne typhus. This is caused by body lice infected with *Rickettsia prowazeki* living intimate contact with humans. Here the initial septicaemic illness is followed by a diffuse purpuric rash; tetracycline 500 mg q.d.s. is the most effective drug.

Tick typhus. A group of rickettsial disease transmitted to humans by the bite of an infected tick, this may afflict hunters as well as the underprivileged. Some varieties produce an initial eschar at the site of the bite, and all are then followed by a headache, fever and petechial rash. They respond briskly to tetracycline 500 mg q.d.s.

(c) Recent travel may be relevant, particularly if it has been to recognised infectious areas.

(d) Your patient may be aware of recent exposure to infection, or a close contact may have a similar illness, which may even have been diagnosed.

(e) Prior surgery or trauma should alert you to the possibility of associated infection.

(f) A menstruating woman using tampons may have the toxic shock syndrome caused by a staphylococcal exotoxin. Antibiotics do not appear to help, but it is reasonable to give flucloxacillin.

(g) Diarrhoea, sometimes bloody, following a course of antibiotics suggests *Clostridium difficile* infection (see p. 122). Sigmoidoscopic appearances are characteristic.

(h) Previous immunisation may be of relevance, if only to exclude those illnesses from which your patient ought to have been protected.

4) You may, however, be faced with a patient with a severe pyrexial illness without any clear localising or associated features. Worldwide, the two major problems here are typhoid (see p. 284) and malaria (see p. 281), and should be considered in every seriously ill pyrexial patient.

Virally induced influenza-like syndromes can simulate these two diseases, but viraemias do not usually give rise to rigors or the same degree of prostration as these more serious conditions.

Many of the conditions mentioned in (3) above can give a septicaemic picture, but the presence of discriminatory symptoms and signs should help you decide between the various causes.

(5) There are non-infectious causes of acute pyrexia. Some have already been mentioned (see (5), p. 271) and are usually easily excluded. In addition:

(i)   adverse reactions to drugs can produce a fever, again the circumstances usually indicate the diagnosis;

(ii) tumours, immunological disorders, chronic infections such as tuberculosis and infective endocarditis, and many other inflammatory diseases such as sarcoid, can produce fever. These conditions do not usually present acutely, assuming major importance only in the investigation of pyrexia of unknown origin.[1]

(6) Discussion of the causes of pyrexia in immunocompromised patients is beyond the scope of this book.

INVESTIGATIONS

Your aim is to identify the specific causal organism as quickly and simply as possible; only in this way will you be able to offer rational therapy.

(1) Take a specimen of urine, sputum, stool, pus, or a swab from any relevant sites, for culture before you begin any antibiotics. Immediate gram staining of this material should be carried out. This will often give you a vivid demonstration of the correctness of your diagnosis.

(2) Take blood cultures, three from different sites is reasonable. Anaerobic cultures should be set up, and you should ask your bacteriologist to let you have a preliminary result in 12–24 h.

(3) Examine the urine for cells, blood and protein, the presence of which will suggest a urinary tract infection.

(4) Take a chest x-ray.

(5) Do a full blood count and stain a blood film, which may show the following.

(i)   Malarial parasites or trypanosomes.

(ii) A lymphocytosis with atypical mononuclear cells, suggestive of mononucleosis.

(iii) An absolute neutrophilia, suggesting a bacterial infection. Typhoid and brucellosis are exceptions, as both are associated with a low white blood count ($<5 \times 10^9/mm^3$). Viral infections do not raise the white cell count.

   (iv) A normochromic normocytic anaemia may suggest haemolysis, common in malaria, or that you are dealing with a more chronic process.

6) If there is any suggestion of meningism, perform a lumbar puncture (see p. 328).
7) Liver function tests are seldom immediately helpful. If you suspect focal intra-abdominal pathology, an abdominal ultrasound is the easiest and quickest way of confirming this; it is anyway a very useful investigation in seeking the cause of occult sepsis.
8) Take blood for serological investigations. These only assume importance retrospectively, as you have to demonstrate a four-fold rise in titre to confirm a particular infection.

REATMENT OF ACUTE PYREXIAL ILLNESS

1) Your clinical examination and preliminary investigations will nearly always suggest the most likely diagnosis, which can then be treated appropriately.
2) Difficulty arises when, despite your best endeavours, you do not have a clear idea of the likely cause of the pyrexia. You have several options.

   (i)   Treat with broad-spectrum antibiotics, as for bacterial shock (see p. 309). This is a reasonable course of action if your patient is poorly perfused, is toxic with rigors, or has evidence of organ failure (see p. 295).

   (ii) Adopt a wait-and-see policy, examining your patient repeatedly and being guided by clinical developments and the results of your investigations. This is the course that we usually adopt.

   (iii) In anyone who has been to a malarious area, especially if there is doubt about the validity of your blood smear, give chloroquine or quinine (see p. 282).

   (iv) In anyone from an area where typhoid is shown to be a prominent problem, give chloramphenicol alone (see p. 285).

In practice, the course you adopt will depend on your perception of w ill your patient is, and the facilities available to you, modified as cessary in the light of clinical developments and the result of vestigations.

REFERENCE

1   Jacoby G. A., Swartz M. N. (1973). Fever of undetermir
     origin. *N. Engl. J. Med.*; **289:** 1407.

Malaria [2]

Malaria due to any of the *Plasmodium* species is, worldwide, one of the commonest causes of an acute pyrexial illness. It often administers the *coup de grâce* to an individual already primarily debilitated and anaemic from a combination of previous infections and malnutrition. Moreover, *Plasmodium falciparum* can give rise to dire complications in previously healthy individuals as follows.

Cerebral malaria. Definitions vary, but this is usually taken to mean a severe encephalopathy with or without focal neurological signs in a patient with acute falciparum infection. The pathogenesis is probably a clogging of small intracerebral blood vessels by parasitised and haemolysed blood cells.

Blackwater fever (malarial haemoglobinuria). This involves massive intravascular haemolysis leading to jaundice and/or acute renal failure. Again, the pathogenesis is obscure; it may occur in the absence of parasitaemia, and is thus presumed to be an immunological response to the parasite.

DIAGNOSIS

(1) Diagnosis of malarial infection depends primarily on seeing parasites in a blood smear. Because the intensity of parasitaemia can vary from hour to hour, several serial blood smears should be examined before abandoning the search. But it is uncommon for a second smear to be positive if no parasites are seen in the initial one.

(2) There is usually a normochromic normocytic anaemia, normal or low white blood count, and the platelet count is frequently reduced to around $100 \times 10^9/l$. This last is presumably due to platelet consumption, but a full blown disseminated intravascular coagulation (DIC) is very uncommon.

(3) Hypoglycaemia may contribute to the coma of malaria, particularly in those treated with quinine. This should always be looked for, and treated with i.v. 10% dextrose infusions (see overleaf).[3]

(4) Malaria can be confused with many other acute pyrexial ill nesses. An approach to this problem is outlined on p. 278.

MANAGEMENT

(1) The mainstay has been oral chloroquine 0.6 g given immedi ately, followed by 0.3 g 6 h later and 0.3 g daily for 2 days. Th i.m. route is an alternative if faced with persistent vomiting

(2) However, the emergence of chloroquine-resistant strains ha: in a variety of localities, forced an alternative regimen, wit quinine, pyrimethamine and a sulphonamide. Quinine dihyd rochloride is given first with a loading infusion of 20 mg/kg i 500 ml of 5% dextrose infused over 4 h. This is followed b 10 mg/kg doses every 8 h given as infusions of 250 ml of 5% dextrose over 4 h. Quinidine may be used as an alternative. It : used similarly as a loading dose (15 mg base/kg), followed b infusions of 7.5 mg base/kg every 8 h. The infusions may b discontinued when the patient can take by mouth. A side-effe of both drugs is hypoglycaemia secondary to induced insuli release. This should be looked for regularly—if necessary beir controlled by the use of 10% dextrose rather than 5%. Th course is continued for 10 days.

(3) In addition, and starting concurrently, pyrimethamine 25 m b.d. is given for 3 days, plus a sulphonamide such as su phadiazine 2 g initially followed by 0.5 g 6-hourly for 5 day:

(4) Anaemia should be treated on its merits by blood transfusio In desperately ill patients with over 10% of red blood ce parasitised, exchange transfusion should be considered.

(5) As mentioned above, the pathogenesis of cerebral malaria obscure. However, cerebral oedema does not play a significar part.[1] Dexamethasone seems to prolong coma in survivors : well as exposing them to the risks of steroid therapy. It has r beneficial effect on mortality.[4]

(6) Having given antimalarials, the treatment of cerebral malaria as for the unconscious patient (see p. 323).

(7) Renal failure in blackwater fever is treated along the usual lin (see p. 144).

(8) Pulmonary oedema, due to leaky capillaries (the ARDS, see 91), occurs in a few patients with severe falciparum malari You must be alert to this possibility. Management is as for oth causes of the ARDS (see p. 92).

REFERENCES

1   Looareesuwan S., Warrell D. A., White N. J. *et al.* (1983). Do patients with cerebral malaria have cerebral oedema? *Lancet*; **i:** 434.

2   Peters W., Hall A. P. (1985). The treatment of severe falciparum malaria. *Br. Med. J.*; **291:** 1146.

3   Phillips R. E. *et al.* (1986). Hypoglycaemia and anti-malarial drugs: quinidine and release of insulin. *Br. Med. J.*; **292:** 1319.

4   Warrell D. A., Looareesuwan S. *et al.* (1982). Dexamethasone proves deleterious in cerebral malaria. *N. Engl. J. Med.*; **306:** 313.

Typhoid [2,4]

DIAGNOSIS

(1) Typhoid, due in 95% of cases to infection with the gram-negative motile rod *Salmonella typhi*, is a leading cause of acute pyrexial illness in underdeveloped countries. The initial symptoms (first phase of the disease) are non-specific and 'flu' like stepwise increase in fever, headache, malaise, anorexia, cough, sore throat and musculoskeletal aches; 10% of patients have associated gastroenteritis. At this stage 90% of patients will have positive blood cultures. Positive stool cultures (in 80%) and urine cultures (in 25%) occur during the second phase of the illness.

(2) The second phase, that of the established disease, begins 2-3 weeks after ingestion of the organism. It is here that the widely known but seldom seen rose-red spots occur; more reliably these patients have bronchitis, lymphadenopathy, splenomegaly, occasionally hepatomegaly, a relative bradycardia, constipation and typhoid stupor. Stupor describes the characteristic mental anergy, which may progress to frank confusion and coma, which is the hallmark of the toxic encephalopathy related to typhoid. Ileal perforation can occur in this phase of the disease.

(3) Occasionally, patients present with the late complications of the disease, either metastatic spread to any site, or immune complex deposition responsible for the glomerulonephritis and probably myocarditis.

(4) So typhoid usually presents as an acute febrile illness. It may present as an emergency in one of three guises.

    (i)   Deteriorating consciousness progressing to coma.

    (ii)   Intestinal perforation. Pain in the right lower quadrant the commonest initial sign, followed by signs of localised or generalised peritonitis. Abdominal x-ray should reveal free air.

    (iii) Intestinal haemorrhage. Macroscopic bleeding occurs not infrequently—massive haemorrhage is fortunately rare signalled by a sudden fall in arterial pressure and temperature.

284

(5) Most but not all patients will achieve at least a fourfold rise in antibodies to O antigen (the Widal test), but this is an unreliable diagnostic pointer, particularly in communities in which salmonella infections are endemic.[3]

(6) Ninety per cent of patients have a normal or low white blood count, and most have a normochromic normocytic anaemia. Jaundice is uncommon, but mild abnormalities of liver enzymes are present in 40% of patients.[1]

(7) In the early stages, typhoid may be confused with many other acute pyrexial illnesses. An approach to the differential diagnosis is outlined on p. 278.

MANAGEMENT

If the diagnosis is suspected, the patient should be isolated and barrier nursed.

(1) Take blood for full blood count, electrolytes and urea and liver function tests. Take three blood cultures and send urine and faecal specimens for bacteriology.

(2) The drug of choice is chloramphenicol. Give 50 mg/kg per day in divided doses 6-hourly, orally if possible, i.v. if not, for 2 weeks.

(3) Coma in typhoid has been assumed to be due to a combination of toxaemia, inanition and fluid and electrolyte derangement. Treatment therefore depends on chemotherapy and ensuring appropriate volume replacement.

(4) If a large perforation is suspected, a laparotomy should be carried out. These patients are obviously not ideal surgical candidates. Careful attention to volume replacement with a CVP line will maximise their chances (p. 343). It may be possible to temporise with bowel rest and volume replacement, with small perforations, since these may self-seal.

(5) Intestinal haemorrhage is treated with blood replacement in the usual way (p. 106).

REFERENCES

1 Hoffman T. A. *et al.* (1975). Waterborne typhoid fever in Dade County, Florida. Clinical and therapeutic evaluation of 105 bacteraemic patients. *Am. J. Med.*; **59**: 481.

2   Hook E. W. (1984). Typhoid fever today. *N. Engl. J. Med.*;
     310: 116.
3   Reynolds D. W. *et al.* (1970). Diagnostic specificity of Widal's
     reaction for typhoid fever. *J. Am. Med. Assoc.*; **214:** 2197.
4   Rubin H. (1983). Enteric fever (case report). *N. Engl. J. Med.*;
     309: 600.

General clinical problems

The uncontrolled and potentially hostile patient

Sudden onset of mental deterioration must be considered an emergency. It constitutes one of the severest tests of clinical skills.

DIAGNOSIS

The following conditions must always be borne in mind.

(1) Cerebral hypoxia (poor perfusion or poor oxygenation).
(2) Infection—any, but particularly meningitis, encephalitis, pneumonia (especially pneumococcal) and septicaemia.
(3) Any pain or discomfort (commonly urinary retention) in a patient already seriously ill.
(4) Drugs—the following most frequently: barbiturates (especially in the elderly), amphetamines, monoamine oxidase inhibitors, atropine, corticosteroids, anti-Parkinsonism drugs, and ephedrine. Almost every drug has been implicated at some time.
(5) An intracranial space-occupying lesion, e.g. tumour, abscess or haematoma (extradural, subdural or intracerebral).
(6) Hypoglycaemia or, more rarely, hyperglycaemia.
(7) Alcohol—either its excess or its sudden withdrawal (see p. 292).
(8) Complex partial seizures, such as may occur in temporal lobe epilepsy.
(9) Myxoedema (see p. 176).
(10) Thyrotoxicosis (see p. 179).
(11) Systemic lupus erythematosus.
(12) Deficiency of thiamine (Wernicke's encephalopathy—external ophthalmoplegia, ataxia and confusion), nicotinamide and vitamin B_{12}.
(13) Hypo- or hypernatraemia.
(14) Hypokalaemia.
(15) Hepatic pre-coma (see p. 130).
(16) Hypo- and hypercalcaemia (see pp. 185, 182).
(17) Acute porphyria.

Two or more of these may occur together. Any may be exacerbated by anaemia, hypotension or pre-existing chronic dementia.

MANAGEMENT

(1) This involves consideration of the above causes. As a routine you must ask for:

  (i)   haemoglobin and PCV;
  (ii)   electrolytes and urea;
  (iii) blood sugar;
  (iv)   blood calcium;
  (v)   blood gases;
  (vi)   skull x-ray;
  (vii) liver function tests, including a prothrombin time;
  (viii) blood culture;
  (ix)   consider a lumbar puncture;

and take a careful drug history.

(2) Confusion is always worse at night. Disorientation may be helped by an easily visible clock, a familiar nurse and a light.

(3) Never attempt to sedate an uncontrolled patient without due consideration of the cause; it may make the situation worse and it may be fatal. If sedation is vital or is deemed unharmful, give chlorpromazine (50–100 mg i.m.) initially or phenobarbitone 100 mg i.m. or diazepam 10 mg i.v.

  If the above are ineffective, give either:

  (i)   chlormethiazole (see p. 292); or
  (ii)   a cocktail of haloperidol 20 mg, kemadrin 20 mg, and promethazine (sparine) 100 mg, all i.m. and drawn up in the same syringe.

This rarely fails to bring peace to the patient and his attendants. Never give paraldehyde to a confused but conscious patient as the pain provides considerable force and direction for the structure of his delusions. It goes without saying that your verbal or pharmacological attempts to calm the patient must not be attended by any hint of aggression. It not only betrays lack of insight on your part, it may also be the only facet of your relationship to be grasped by the patient— and is therefore disastrous.

Acute psychoses

DIAGNOSIS

The clinical picture may be very similar to some of the conditions described on p. 289, and if in doubt you must do at least (1) (i)–(vi) on p. 290. In addition, sudden medical or surgical illness may provoke an acute psychosis in a sufficiently susceptible patient.

A history of previous mental illness may therefore be present. A helpful point of distinction between an acute psychosis and a toxic confusional state is that in the former the sensorium is clear, although the content of thought is disordered.

Consider the following.

(1) Puerperal psychosis.
(2) Acute schizophrenia. This usually presents a characteristic mixture of disorders of thinking and feelings, with hallucinations and disorders of conduct. It closely resembles the picture of amphetamine psychosis.
(3) Acute depression. Delusions and hallucinations are usually of a self-deprecatory nature. Hypochondriasis, suicidal ruminations and a tendency to depersonalisation may be evident.
(4) Acute mania. Elation combines characteristically with easily provoked irritability. The patient talks rapidly, jumping from one subject to another.
(5) Acute hysterical episodes. Overtones of acting and self-dramatisation may be apparent. Even when at his most violent, the patient rarely injures himself.

MANAGEMENT

Management of these patients involves the following.

(1) Achieving, if at all possible, some kind of contact with the patient, if only to establish yourself as a harmless and possibly helpful comrade.
(2) Consideration of the general principles as outlined in sections (2) and (3) on p. 290.
(3) Initiating the treatment of specific psychiatric syndromes.
(4) Psychiatric consultation, which should be sought as soon as possible.

Toxic confusional state due to acute alcohol withdrawal—delirium tremens[2,3]

Acute withdrawal from alcohol causes a characteristic toxic confusional state which, if uncontrolled, may be fatal.

DIAGNOSIS

(1) Delirium tremens (DTs) usually occurs in a patient who has been withdrawn suddenly from alcohol after a binge lasting at least 2 weeks, and often considerably longer.

(2) The characteristic symptoms are tremulousness, apprehension, disorientation in time and place, and visual, tactile and auditory hallucinations. In addition, insomnia, nausea and vomiting and motor incoordination may be present.

(3) These symptoms usually begin within hours of withdrawal, and are maximal from about 24 to 48 h. Their occurrence should be anticipated in persons known to be heavy drinkers.

(4) Excessive intake of alcohol may also give rise to cirrhosis, cardiomyopathy and various neurological syndromes such as peripheral neuropathy due to vitamin deficiency, chronic cerebellar disease and Wernicke's encephalopathy. Thus, DTs may be superimposed on an already debilitated patient.

(5) There is a substantial and rather unpredictable variability in the severity of the symptoms of withdrawal. About 80% of patients get mild symptoms, 14% moderate trouble and 6% progress to full-blown DTs.

MANAGEMENT

Non-specific

(1) It is very important to establish contact with the patient who is frightened, disorientated and frequently aggressive.

(2) Thiamine 50 mg i.v. and 50 mg i.m. should always be given

before starting a dextrose infusion, thereby avoiding the possibility of precipitating Wernicke's encephalopathy in a susceptible patient.

Specific

(1) The aim of treatment is the induction of light sleep sufficient to control symptoms, whilst leaving vital functions unimpaired. Drugs to achieve this end are best given orally, but may have to be given i.v.

(2) Chlormethiazole (Heminevrin) is the drug of choice.[1] The dose required to achieve (1) above ranges between 4.0 g/day and 10.0 g/day. It needs to be reviewed daily, the highest dose generally being needed 24–48 h after alcohol withdrawal.

   Patients generally do not need this drug after the seventh day. If oral administration is impossible, i.v. chlormethiazole may be given. Give a loading dose of 30–50 ml of a 0.8% solution over 3–5 min to induce sleep, and continue an infusion of this concentration at 0.5–1.0 ml/min, adjusting the rate to the minimum dose required to keep the patient just sleeping lightly. Usually, 500–1000 ml are needed in the first 6–12 h. If it is used in this way for a maximum of 12–18 h, chlormethiazole is a safe drug. Side-effects, which are dose related, are respiratory depression, hypotension and supraventricular tachycardia culminating in respiratory arrest. For this reason you should not continue the infusion for longer than 18 h without first measuring chlormethiazole levels.

(3) Chlordiazepoxide, either orally or i.v., in sufficient dosage necessary to induce light sleep, may be used as an alternative to chlormethiazole. Start with 40 mg 4-hourly and increase to 100 mg 2-hourly if necessary.

(4) Although the tremulousness, fever, tachycardia and hallucinations subside over 3–4 days, there may be an interval over 1–2 weeks before full return to the patient's previous mental state. This interval is characterised by a lack of concentration and intermittent disorientation and agitated confusion. The latter is best treated with haloperidol 10 mg i.m. hourly as necessary (with a maximum of 60 mg/24 h). This may precipitate dystonic reactions which may be relieved by benztropine 2 mg i.m.

(5) Promazine derivatives should not be used, because of their hepatoxic effect, and opiates should be avoided as they may cause respiratory depression in persons with liver damage.

(6) The possibility of cirrhosis, heart failure and neurological disease induced by alcohol should be considered during examination of the patient, as these may need treating also. To this end, the following investigations should be made as soon as possible: chest x-ray, ECG, liver function tests and serum proteins, full blood picture and ESR, serum folate, electrolytes and blood urea.

   Remember, all this is only first aid and your psychiatric colleagues should be involved as early as possible.

REFERENCES

1   Hollister L. E. *et al*. (1972). Treatment of acute alcohol withdrawal with chlormethiazole. *Dis. Nerv. Sys*.; **33:** 247.
2   Leader (1981). Management of alcohol withdrawal symptoms. *Br. Med. J.*; **282:** 502.
3   Lerner W. D., Fallon H. J. (1985). The alcohol withdrawal syndrome. *N. Engl. J. Med.*; **313:** 951.

The poorly perfused patient [1,2,4,5]

DIAGNOSIS

A persistently low arterial pressure (systolic <70 mmHg) is of itself life threatening, but a lesser degree of hypotension does not matter unless there is also evidence of inadequate tissue perfusion, when it should always be regarded as a medical emergency. This combination also provides a working definition of shock.

An alternative, perhaps more apposite, definition of shock is the sensation experienced by the house officer after he has been looking after a deteriorating patient for 3 h!

Poor tissue perfusion is most easily seen when it affects the following sites.

(1) The brain—mental confusion.
(2) The extremities (including the nose)—which are cold, pale, moist and mottled with peripheral cyanosis and collapsed veins.
(3) The kidneys—the minimal acceptable urine flow rate is 0.5 ml/kg per hour. If it is less than this, renal hypoperfusion is likely to be present. If the temperature of the extremities falls much below that of the central temperature (as measured on a rectal thermometer), this implies poor tissue perfusion and a fall in the glomerular filtration rate is also likely.
(4) The coronary arteries—this may be the cause of arrhythmias and also of impaired myocardial contractility.

The shock syndrome can arise from four basic causes.

(1) Cardiogenic (more accurately, primary pump failure). The main causes here are:

    (i)   myocardial infarction (see p. 10) and/or heart failure from any cause.
    (ii)   cardiac arrhythmias, particularly Stokes–Adams attacks and ventricular tachycardias (see p. 32).

(2) Decreased circulating volume leading to hypovolaemia. The main causes here are:

    (i)   salt and water depletion as in severe diarrhoea and vomiting, heat exhaustion and diabetic and Addisonian crisis;

   (ii)   haemorrhage (see p. 106);
   (iii) anaphylaxis (see p. 305).

(3) Decreased vascular resistance, leading to abnormalities of distribution. Here there is a mismatch between the vascular bed and the circulating blood volume from the outset. The main causes here are:

   (i)   septic shock (see p. 307);
   (ii) barbiturate and other overdoses.

(4) Obstructive. Here the venous return to the right or left atrium is compromised. The main causes here are:

   (i)   cardiac tamponade (see p. 60);
   (ii) mediastinal shift: this is usually due to massive pulmonary collapse (see p. 84), a large pleural effusion (see p. 89) overhasty relief of a large pleural effusion (see p. 89), or pneumothorax (see p. 80);
   (iii) pulmonary embolism (see p. 47);
   (iv) dissecting aneurysm (see p. 58).

Any of the above causes, if sufficiently prolonged or severe, may cause a reduced cardiac output and high peripheral resistance. The ensuing poor tissue perfusion causes a profound acidosis which dilates the precapillary arterioles, but not the postcapillary venules. This causes stagnation of blood within the capillaries which both exacerbates cellular hypoxia and, because of damage to the capillary walls, causes leakage of crystalloid and colloid from the vascular compartment. Further, in shock the entire capillary bed is involved so that the capacitance of the vascular compartment is increased.

Thus, the initiating sequence of events in shock is compounded by

   (i)   stasis of blood within the capillaries;
   (ii) extravasation of crystalloid and colloid from damaged capillaries;
   (iii) increase in capacitance of the circulatory system.

The result of all this is a serious mismatch between the effective blood volume (much reduced) and the capacitance of the vascular compartment (increased). This mismatch is reflected clinically in the poor tissue perfusion, hypotension, tachycardia and lowered CVP which characterise shock. Prompt treatment is intended to reverse the above outlined sequence, thereby preventing the inexorable progression which will otherwise ensue.

An understanding of the pathogenesis of shock is essential to its proper management, which is further outlined below.

MANAGEMENT

Monitoring and investigations

Patients with shock in whom aggressive therapy is warranted need to be looked after in an intensive care unit. Basic monitoring should include the following.

(1) Arterial pressure. This is measured by an intra-arterial catheter which will not only give you a continuous readout, but can be used to obtain arterial blood for blood gas measurements.

(2) Pulse and respiratory rate.

(3) Temperature. You need to measure core and toe temperatures. Moderate pyrexia is a valuable asset in combating infection (most obviously in the lizard, which, when ill, seeks a warm niche in which to induce a temperature), and is also, of course, a frequent pointer to infection. In addition, skin temperature is a reflection of the peripheral blood flow. Normally the gradient between core and periphery is 3°C, whereas in shock, the peripheral temperature (most conveniently measured on the big toe) is often only 2°C above the ambient temperature. A closing of the core–peripheral temperature gap is valuable evidence of improvement.

(4) Central venous pressure and pulmonary artery occlusion pressure (PAOP). These measure the right- and left-sided filling pressures respectively, and so can be used to guide your fluid replacement (see p. 343).

(5) A continuous ECG recording should be established.

(6) Urinary output. As mentioned above, this is an important indicator of tissue perfusion. You may also need to test the urinary osmolality (see p. 139) to assess whether renal function is adequate.

(7) Investigations. You will need to do a Hb, white cell count, platelet count, and clotting studies if there is any evidence of bleeding (see below). Take arterial blood for gases and pH, and venous blood for electrolytes (including Ca^{2+}, Mg^{2+} PO_4), liver function tests and urea. You may need to measure lactate (see p. 168). Blood cultures should be taken so that you can prescribe antibiotics intelligently (see p. 309).

(8) Colloid osmotic pressure (COP). Traditionally, we have equated serum albumin with COP. We now realise that this is not a very satisfactory equation. However, it is now possible to measure COP directly, the normal being 25 mmHg. In accordance with Starling's law, raising the intravascular COP will increase the amount of fluid in the intravascular compartment and so will be useful in assessing how much of which fluid, particularly colloid, you should give. As this is one of the major unresolved problems in the treatment of shock (see below), you should strive to get access to COP measurements. While awaiting this technological advance, it is better to use the total protein rather than the albumin as an indirect measure of COP

(9) Daily chest x-rays. These are desirable, if only to make sure you have not produced a pneumothorax inserting your central lines!

(10) Transcutaneous O_2 and CO_2. Monitoring of these is emerging as a useful guide to tissue perfusion and oxygenation, and may be available to you.

Specific

These measures are directed towards removing the cause, which is usually apparent from the history and examination. This is, however, not usually sufficient, further measures being required to correct tissue perfusion.

Non-specific

(1) You must ensure that your patient has a clear airway. If there doubt in your mind, or if the airway is at risk, intubate the patient.

(2) Restoring the circulating volume. Effective restoration of the circulating volume is the single most important measure in reversing shock.

The questions to be answered are how much of which fluid will be required?

(i) *How much?* As outlined above, many factors contribute to the hypovolaemia of shock. Thus the volume of fluid required to restore perfusion is always greater than any fluid loss (which is, anyway, difficult to measure). Improving tissue perfusion is evidenced by a warming of the extremities, increasing renal flow and disappearance of mental confusion. The amount of fluid to achieve this is best assessed by serial CVP readings (see p. 343). A CVP line is thus mandatory in the proper treatment of shock, but of course fluid replacement should begin immediately, and not wait on the placement of the line, which may be difficult. Insertion of a pulmonary artery flotation catheter (see p. 347), enabling you to record pulmonary wedge pressure and cardiac output, can also be very helpful in assessing fluid requirements, and is being used more frequently in the monitoring of shock patients.

(ii) *Which fluids?* Irrespective of the cause of shock, both crystalloids and colloids are lost, and both require replacement. The circumstances in which shock occurs will obviously determine the ratio of colloid to crystalloid used, but as a general rule, one-half to three-quarters of the necessary volume should be as crystalloid, and the rest as colloid, although controversy over the exact ratio abounds. Crystalloids should be given initially as normal saline, as salt replacement has first priority. However, in overall terms there is usually more water than salt lost, thus it is reasonable to give one-third of the overall crystalloid replacement as 5% dextrose.

Colloid replacement can be as albumin, plasma or one of the artificial plasma expanders, such as dextran or Haemaccel. Dextran is cheap, readily available and free from the risk of hepatitis, and has, as an additional bonus, an antithrombotic property (see (4) below). However, it does tend to block the reticuloendothelial system, an undesirable property. Dextran 70 in saline, in a dose of no more than 1000 ml/24 h, is still being regarded by some as the colloid of choice. Dextran 40, whilst having the theoretical advantage of reducing viscosity, can cause renal failure; we do not use it. If colloid additional to the dextrans proves to be necessary, plasma may be used. In hypovolaemic cardiogenic shock, or in any other circumstances where saline infusion is undesirable, dextran made up in dextrose can be used. As dextrans cause rouleaux formation, blood must be taken for cross-matching before they are infused. Haemaccel, a colloid made from degraded gelatine, does not have antithrombotic properties. It does not cause cross-matching difficulties, and is said to have renal protective effects, so we use it in preference to dextran. We do not use more than 2000 ml in any single shock episode.

The purpose of giving colloid is to raise the intravascular oncotic pressure, and so entrain fluid into the vascular compartment. Normal colloid osmotic pressure is 25 mmHg, and research is underway to assess which colloid solution is best at raising the intravascular osmotic pressure. This will mean that in the near future we should be able to advance a more rational colloid replacement policy.

In haemorrhagic shock, blood will be required in addition to the above fluids. It is probably desirable to transfuse the patient to a haemoglobin of around 11 g/100 ml. Higher than this does not materially alter O_2 delivery, but does have the disadvantage of increasing viscosity. The blood that you give may obviate the need for any other colloid. The perfluorochemicals (O_2-carrying substances) are being evaluated as substitutes for blood. Their role is not yet defined.[3]

(3) Reversing hypoxia. The importance of ensuring a clear airway has already been stressed. Use of high (40–60%) concentrations of O_2 will improve the PaO_2 and ensure maximal saturation of haemoglobin. This may prevent some cell damage. This O_2 concentration can be achieved by most commercially available face masks, using O_2 flow rates of about 10 l/min. Assisted ventilation may be required, particularly if shock lung occurs (see p. 91). The use of hyperbaric O_2 is still experimental.

(4) Reducing arteriolar constriction. Arteriolar constriction should reverse when the cardiac output and arterial pressure are restored to normal with your fluid replacement. If, however, fluid replacement alone is not sufficient, you should use either of the following.

    (i)   Beta-adrenergic agents, such as dopamine and dobutamine.[3] At low infusion rates (<5 μg/kg per min) dopamine induces selective vasodilatation of the renal, cerebral, coronary and mesenteric circulations. At slightly higher doses (5–20 μg/kg per min), it increases the force but not the rate of myocardial contraction (i.e. is inotropic not chronotropic). Its maximal effect is said to triple the heart force. It is thus the agent of choice in shock, once you are satisfied that volume repletion is adequate (see p. 343).

        Dobutamine (2.5–10 μg/kg per min) is more strongly

inotropic than dopamine, but does not have dopamine's vasodilator properties. Using the two together makes good sense, as we have outlined in the section on cardiogenic shock (p. 16).

If these are not available, or do not work, use isoprenaline. Put 2 mg of isoprenaline in 500 ml of 5% dextrose and give the infusion sufficiently fast to raise the systolic arterial pressure to about 95 mmHg. If this is ineffective or leads to a large volume of fluid being infused, double or treble the concentration.

All these are preferable to metaraminol (aramine), which has both alpha-mimetic and beta-mimetic properties and may increase the arterial pressure at some expense to tissue perfusion.

Noradrenaline and methoxamine should not be used. They constrict arterioles and further decrease tissue perfusion. Their use is therefore illogical, and in practice is rarely successful.

(ii) Alpha-adrenergic blocking agents, the use of which has been largely superseded by dopamine and dobutamine. These reduce arteriolar constriction. The agents most commonly used are phenoxybenzamine, phentolamine, chlorpromazine and nitroprusside. They can cause a disastrous fall in arteral pressure unless the expanded circulating volume is taken up by infusing fluid, preferably blood, plasma, dextran 70 or Haemaccel. It is essential for the CVP and/or the PCWP to be at the upper limit of the normal range before these drugs are given. Infuse phenoxybenzamine 10–15 mg in 100 ml of 5% dextrose over 2 h, or phentolamine at a rate of 0.5–1 mg/min, or chlorpromazine 5 mg i.v. every 15 min to a maximum of 20 mg. Give nitroprusside as outlined on p. 45. As the drug is given, the CVP will probably fall, together with the PCWP and arterial pressure. The CVP and or PCWP must be maintained within the upper half of the normal range by further infusions of fluid. This ensures adequate venous return and cardiac output.

5) Glucocorticoids. In pharmacological doses they may have some inotropic effect on the heart, cause arteriolar dilatation, and may protect against the development of shock lung. Their role and action are not clear, and the studies that there are do not support their use. We do not use them as a routine. However,

some authorities give methyl prednisolone 30 mg/kg i.v. over 20 min; the dose may be repeated once, 6 h later. This sort of dose does not suppress the pituitary–adrenal axis and so can be stopped abruptly.

(6) Increasing myocardial contractility. The reason for myocardial depression in shock is not clear, although certain products of cell necrosis have been implicated. You should attempt to reverse this depression with adrenergic agents, with the correction of the acidosis, and by ensuring that your patient has correct levels of all the other electrolytes, including K^+, Mg^{2+}, Ca^{2+}, PO_4^{2-}. It may also be of benefit to digitalise the patient (see p. 16).

(7) Reversing acidosis. As acidosis has a well-recognised negative inotropic effect, its correction is important, and is usually achieved by restoring tissue perfusion. However, if the pH is below 7.1, it is reasonable to give small quantities of bicarbonate. Theoretically the bicarbonate deficit (mmol) is given by (body weight (kg) $\times$ 3/5) $\times$ (25 $-$ serum HCO_3 mmol/l). Give half this amount and remeasure the arterial pH before deciding whether to give more.

(8) More controversial is the use of heparin. Enzymes released from damaged cells convert fibrinogen to fibrin, thus creating a state of disseminated intravascular coagulation (DIC) which may further impair tissue perfusion. The evidence for DIC is bleeding tendency with low platelets, raised prothrombin time (PT) and kaolin cephalin time (KCT), low fibrinogen titres and raised fibrin degradation products. There may be fragmented red cells on the blood film. A reasonable bedside test for the presence of DIC is as follows.

Take blood into a plain tube and keep this at 37°C (98.6°F) by holding it in your hand or putting it in your pocket. Invert it at 30 s intervals. Normal blood should clot within 2–3 min. Failure to do this is good evidence for DIC.

These abnormalities are often reversed when the underlying cause of shock is corrected; there is no good evidence that the use of heparin increases survival. Fresh frozen plasma, which supplies all the major clotting factors, should be given as a part of the fluids required to support the circulation. If, after the underlying disorder is corrected, bleeding persists with a low plasma fibrinogen level (<1.0 g/l) and a low platelet count ($<40 \times 10^9/l$), fibrinogen concentrate and fresh platelet concentrates may be required.

REFERENCES

1   Davies J. M. (1982). Cardiovascular problems. *Hosp. Update*; **Nov:** 1359.
2   Houston M. C. (1984). Shock, Diagnosis and management. *Arch. Intern. Med.*; **144:** 1433.
3   Leader (1986). Blood substitutes. Has the right solution been found? *Lancet*; **i:** 717.
4   Ledingham I. McA. *et al.* (1982). Prognosis in severe shock. *Br. Med. J.*; **284:** 443.
5   Levine B. S., Coburn J. W. (1984). Magnesium, the mimic/ antagonist of calcium. *N. Engl. J. Med.*; **310:** 1253.

Blood transfusion reactions

A mild reaction consisting of flushing, itching and urticaria is quite common, especially in those with a history of allergic reactions. Their incidence may be reduced by antihistamines, e.g. diphenhydramine (Benadryl) 50 mg orally 1 h before transfusion and 50 mg during it. If wheezing starts to occur or hypotension (which is not due to haemorrhage) develops, the blood should be stopped at once and saved for retesting. Give hydrocortisone 200 mg i.v. or adrenaline 1 : 1000 0.5 ml subcutaneously immediately. Also give an i.v. antihistamine such as diphenhydramine 20 mg i.v.

Acute renal failure as a complication of blood transfusion has been dealt with elsewhere (see p. 140).

Anaphylactic shock [1,2,3]

Never give any drug or vaccine to a patient who says he is allergic to it, even if the evidence is unconvincing.

Do not attempt to obtain the evidence by skin testing. This may be misleading and may occasionally be fatal. Warning signs are flushing, itching and urticaria. However, they may be absent. The symptoms of a more severe attack are wheezing, a feeling of chest constriction, abdominal pain, nausea and vomiting. Circulatory collapse and death may follow.

MANAGEMENT

(1) Give adrenaline 500–1000 µg (0.5–1.0 ml of 1 : 1000) i.m. to combat shock. This dose should be repeated at 15 min intervals until improvement occurs. If your patient is profoundly hypotensive (systolic arterial pressure <80 mmHg), 3–5 ml of 1 : 10 000 solution may be given slowly i.v.

(2) Give diphenhydramine hydrochloride (Benadryl) 20 mg slowly i.v. to counteract the excessive histamine release.

(3) Give hydrocortisone 200 mg i.v. to suppress any further allergic reaction.

(4) Give aminophylline 0.5 g i.v. over 5 min if there is evidence of continuing airways obstruction. Do not forget dyspnoea may also be due to acute laryngeal oedema (see p. 86).

(5) Give 35% O_2 if there is cyanosis.

(6) If there are signs of shock or if there is profound hypotension, establish a CVP line and infuse plasma, dextran 70, Haemaccel or alternating bottles of N saline and 5% dextrose to maintain a CVP in the upper half of the normal range. This is usually sufficient to restore the arterial pressure. If, however, it remains low, it may be necessary to give isoprenaline or dopamine (see p. 300).

REFERENCES

1   Austen K. F. (1974). Systemic anaphylaxis in the human being. *N. Engl. J. Med.*; **291**: 661.

2   Fath J. J., Cerra F. B. (1984). The therapy of anaphylactic shock. *Drug Intell. Clin. Pharmacol*.; **18:** 14.
3   Leader (1981). Treatment of anaphylactic shock. *Br. Med. J*.; **282:** 1011.

Bacterial shock [1,4,5,8,9]

DIAGNOSIS

(1) Bacterial shock occurs when large numbers of either gram-positive or gram-negative bacteria get into the bloodstream. Gram-negative bacteraemia quite often follows surgery to the bowel or instrumentation of the lower urinary tract. The infecting organisms are commonly *Escherichia coli* or other coliforms, and, less commonly, anaerobes or *Pseudomonas aeruginosa.* Gram-positive bacteraemias are often secondary to joint or chest sepsis or drug abuse. The causative organisms are usually staphylococci,[10] streptococci or pneumococci. *Clostridium perfringens (welchii)* septicaemia following abortion is an important special group (see Table 3 for antibiotic sensitivities). A further important subgroup to consider is focal, often trivial staphylococcal infection causing toxic shock encephalopathy. In this group, circulating exotoxins cause multiorgan damage. A significant proportion of cases have been associated with the use of tampons during menstruation. Toxic shock encephalopathy may be distinguished clinically. A characteristic macular erythroderma is followed by desquamation, including the palms and soles, within 2 weeks of onset. Mucous membrane changes, oropharyngeal oedema, ulceration and conjunctivitis develop soon after the fever. Fits may occur. Hypotension is often profound.

(2) The onset of septic shock is usually marked by rigors associated with nausea, vomiting and diarrhoea. Initially the patient is peripherally vasodilated, flushed, pyrexial and hypotensive. Cardiac output is at this stage increased, but as much of the blood is being shunted through arteriovenous communications, the $Pa O_2$ is low and tissue O_2 utilisation is deficient. The situation is peculiar to bacteraemic shock, and accounts for the paradox of an apparently well-perfused patient who is, nonetheless, confused and oliguric. The mortality of this group is about 25%. This state gives way to the classical shock picture of a confused or comatose patient with cold, clammy peripheries, acidosis and a fall in urinary and cardiac output with or without pyrexia. The mortality of this group is at least 60%. Early recognition and energetic treatment of the former

Table 4   Sensitivity of common organisms to various antibiotics

	Staphylococcus aureus (gram +ve coccus)		Pseudomonas aeruginosa (gram –ve rod)	Escherichia coli (gram –ve rod)	Proteus sp. (gram –ve rod)	Bacteroides sp. (gram –ve rod)	Clostridium welchii (gram +ve coccus)	Klebsiella aerobacter sp. (gram –ve rod)	Streptococcus pyogenes (gram +ve coccus)	Streptococcus faecalis (gram +ve coccus)
	Hospital acquired	Non-hospital acquired								
Azlocillin/piperacillin	R	S	SS	S	S	SS	HS	SS	S	S
Ceftazidine/cefotaxime	S	S	S	SS	S	R	S	S	S	R
Chloramphenicol	S	S	R	S	SS	S	S	S	S	S
Aminoglycosides/(gentamicin)	HS	HS	S	S	S	R	R	S	R	R
Benzylpenicillin/erythromycin	R	HS	R	R	R	R	HS	R	HS	S
Metronidazole	R	R	R	R	R	S	S	R	R	R
Flucloxacillin	S	S	R	R	R	R	?	R	S	R

state may forestall the appearance of the latter with consequent saving of life.

MANAGEMENT

In about half the patients, the interval between onset of shock and death is 48 h, and a successful outcome is partially dependent upon the speed with which the following measures are carried out.

(1) Laboratory investigations. Take blood for blood cultures, full blood count, electrolytes, urea, and creatinine, group and cross-match and arterial blood gases. If possible, take three blood cultures each from a different site within ½ h. Take swabs from throat and rectum. Microscope and plate out a clean specimen of urine.

(2) Antibiotics (Table 4).

   (i) Start initial treatment as soon as possible after (**never** before!) culture specimens have been taken.

   (ii) Use a combination of a penicillin plus an aminoglycoside plus metronidazole (see (iii), (iv) and (v) below).

   (iii) Choice of penicillin.

   (a) Benzylpenicillin, in combination with an aminoglycoside, is effective against virtually all gram-positive organisms (penicillinase-producing staphylococci will be dealt with by the aminoglycosides). A suitable penicillin dose for severe infections is 2 mega units i.v. every 6 h.

   (b) If the patient is allergic to penicillin, substitute erythromycin 500–1000 mg i.v. 6-hourly.

   (c) If pseudomonas infection or other resistant gram-negative infection is considered likely, substitute piperacillin (200 mg/kg i.v. 6-hourly) or azlocillin 5 g 8-hourly i.v. for the penicillin.

   (d) Azlocillin is synergistic with gentamicin but these must be given in separate infusions, as they react chemically, inactivating each other. This reaction is only of serious consequence in the bloodstream when renal function is seriously impaired.

   (e) Remember that 15 g of azlocillin contains 33 mmol of Na^+, and so Na^+ administration should be adjusted accordingly.

   (f) If your patient is allergic to penicillin, use ceftazidine 1–4 g i.v. 8-hourly in place of piperacillin or azlocillin.

(iv)   Choice of aminoglycoside.

   (a) Aminoglycosides are highly active against nearly all gram-negative organisms. Gentamicin, 5 mg/kg per day in three divided doses (normally 80 mg 8-hourly) is the aminoglycoside of first choice, unless the patient is known to have poor renal function. If you do use gentamicin when renal function is impaired, the interval between doses must be modified as outlined in Table 5. An alternative way of calculating the dose interval is: serum creatinine (μmol) divided by 15 = approximate dosage interval (h). In every case serum gentamicin levels should be measured daily. You should aim for peak levels (1 h after i.v. or i.m. administration) of 7–12 μg/ml, and trough level (just before the next dose) of 2 μg/ml, and you will have to alter your dose as necessary to achieve this.

   (b) Netilmicin is safer in renal impairment, as it is less ototoxic and nephrotoxic. The usual adult dose is 150 mg b.d. (4–7 mg/kg per day in two divided doses). You should aim at peak levels of 5–12 μg/ml and troughs of less than 3 μg/ml.

   (c) Amikacin. This very expensive aminoglycoside should only be used if organisms resistant to gentamicin and netilmicin have been identified. The usual dose is 15 mg/kg per day in two divided doses.

The interval between doses of both the above will have to be modified along the same lines as gentamicin if your patient has renal impairment.

Table 5   Modification of gentamicin dosage in patients with renal impairment

Blood urea (mmol/l)	Dose (mg) and frequency of administration (for a 70 kg patient)	
7	*80	8-hourly
7–18	*80	12-hourly
18–36	*80	24-hourly
36	*80	48-hourly

*60 mg if patient is below 60 kg weight.

(v)   Metronidazole.[3] This is the agent of choice against anaerobes. As mentioned above, we use it routinely in septic shock, as anaerobic organisms are frequently present. The dose is 500 mg in 100 ml infused over ½h, 8-hourly. Alternatively, give 400 mg orally or 1 g rectally 8-hourly.

(vi) Fusidic acid. If severe staphylococcal infection is strongly suspected, give 500 mg fusidic acid dissolved in 250 ml of N saline and infused over 4 h four times a day.

(vii) Chloramphenicol. This is a highly effective antibiotic whose role has been somewhat eclipsed by the aminoglycosides, and its undoubted, though rare, propensity to cause an idiosyncratic irreversible agranulocytosis. More common is the dose-related, reversible marrow suppression. Neither should stop you using it, in a dose of 50–100 mg/kg body weight i.v. 6-hourly, if the newer antibiotics are not available to you. A usual adult dose would be 1 g 6-hourly.

(3) Fungal infection.[7] Systemic candidiasis often occurs in the setting of a bacterial septicaemia, but seldom causes septic shock on its own. Remember, a positive blood culture is not necessarily indicative of systemic disease, but if you believe there to be a significant candidal infection, the treatment is a combination of (i) and (ii) below.

(i)   Amphotericin B. First give a test dose of 1 mg in 20 ml 5% dextrose. Then, if no adverse reaction occurs, give 0.3 mg/kg on the first day and 0.6 mg/kg on subsequent days.

Renal toxicity is a common problem after a few days therapy and you should temporarily stop the drug if the serum creatinine goes above 200 μmol/l.

Hypokalaemia is another well-recognised complication of amphotericin administration, so check the K^+ regularly.

(ii) Flucytosine. Use a dose of 37.5 mg/kg per 6 h orally if renal function is normal. If the creatinine clearance is between 20 ml/min and 40 ml/min, reduce the dose interval to 12-hourly, and if it is 10–20 ml/min, to 37.5 mg/kg each 24 h.

(iii) Ketoconazole. This broad-spectrum oral antifungal agent is effective in mucocutaneous candidiasis, and in the prophylaxis of candidal infections. The dose is 200–400 mg/day.

(4) The restoration of tissue perfusion and correction of metabolic abnormalities are as detailed on p. 298, but in addition the following factors should be borne in mind.

(i) These patients are particularly prone to hypoxia, and frequently require assisted ventilation to maintain the PaO_2. This should be undertaken in conjunction with your anaesthetic colleagues. Even despite ventilatory assistance, respiratory failure is a frequent mode of death. The lung capillaries appear to become leaky, giving an x-ray appearance of widespread consolidation. This respiratory complication is rather unsatisfactorily labelled shock lung, or the adult respiratory distress syndrome (see p. 91).

(ii) Naloxone may be helpful. Endogenous opioids may be responsible for part of the initial hypotension in bacteraemic shock. Naloxone blocks the action of these endogenous opioids, and its role in shock is being evaluated. Preliminary evidence is that at a dose of 0.4–1.2 mg i.v. it may be useful.[6]

(iii) Endotoxin antibody needs to be considered. The lipopolysaccharide in the outer membrane of gram-negative bacteria is not affected by antibiotics, and is thought to be a major factor in the pathogenesis of bacteraemic shock. A recent trial using antibodies to this lipopolysaccharide showed a greatly increased survival.[7]

REFERENCES

1   Atkins E. (1983). Fever—new perspectives on an old phenomenon. *N. Engl. J. Med.*; **308:** 958.

2   Baumgartner J. D. *et al.* (1985). Prevention of gram negative shock and death in surgical patients by antibody to endotoxin core glycolipid. *Lancet*; **ii:** 59.

3   Goldman P. (1980). Metronidazole. *N. Engl. J. Med.*; **303:** 1212.

4   Kass E. H. (1984). High dose corticosteroids for septic shock. *N. Engl. J. Med.*; **311:** 1178.

5   *Lancet* (1982). Good antimicrobial prescribing. *Lancet*; **ii:** 83.
    (This is the first of a series of articles in the *Lancet* on
    antibiotics.)
6   Leader (1981). Naloxone for septic shock. *Lancet*; **i:** 538.
7   Leader (1983). Fungaemia. *Lancet*; **ii:** 323.
8   Leader (1985). A nasty shock from antibiotics? *Lancet*; **ii:** 594.
9   Ledingham I. McA. (1978). Prospective study of the treatment
    of septic shock. *Lancet*; **i:** 1194.
10 Sheagren J. N. (1984). *Staphylococcus aureus.* The persistent
    pathogen. *N. Engl. J. Med.*; **310:** 1360.

The unconscious patient—coma[1-5]

DIAGNOSIS

Coma is an unarousable lack of awareness. It can also be defined as a rating on the Glasgow coma scale of less than 8. Consciousness depends on interconnections between neurons of the ascending reticular formation of the brainstem, which pass through the diencephalon and ramify with neurons throughout the cerebral cortex. Therefore a depression of consciousness leading to coma can be due either to widespread bilateral cortical involvement or to involvement of the diencephalon or brainstem, as detailed below.

(1) Bilateral and widespread dysfunction of both cerebral hemispheres.
(2) Damage to, or compression of, the activating centres of the brainstem and diencephalon.

33%

(3) Metabolic disturbance involving either of the above regions. It is to be distinguished from: 65%
(4) Psychogenic unresponsiveness. 2%

The pattern and sequencing of neurological abnormality can, to a large extent, distinguish which of these is most likely, thus providing information both as to localisation and cause. Since both these are crucial to management, a careful history from relatives (or other witnesses, including the family practitioner or ambulance driver as necessary) and examination are mandatory.

When examining a comatose patient, you aim to find out the following.

(1) The depth of coma. A convenient way to do this is to use the Glasgow coma scale (see p. 202). The depth of coma should be charted at frequent intervals, and any deterioration should call for immediate reassessment of your patient, if necessary by a more experienced colleague.
(2) The presence of focal lesions. Asymmetrical motor responses are the easiest to identify, and these should already have been detected whilst the depth of coma was being assessed. Asymmetry of the brainstem reflexes is also important in this respect (see part B p. 315 and Table 6).
     The presence of persistent focal lesions implies structural rather than metabolic, causes for coma.

314

(3) The anatomical level of involvement of the neuraxis. Here you must be guided by the patterns of involvement of the brainstem reflexes, the type and rate of respiration, and the pulse rate, as detailed below and in Table 6.

Knowledge of these three basic aspects of coma will help you arrive at a differential diagnosis as discussed in the ensuing parts. In parts A and B below, we give an account of the diagnosis and progression of structural lesions causing coma, and in parts C and D, of metabolic and psychogenic causes of coma. In part E we present a flow diagram illustrating our approach to the management of coma.

Part A: Widespread dysfunction of both cerebral hemispheres

(1) Postictal stupor may, if a history is lacking, cause diagnostic confusion, which fortunately is temporary since the patient will usually rouse within 6 h.

Other causes are more serious and essentially are limited to the following.
(2) Catastrophic intracerebral or intraventricular haemorrhage (see p. 189).
(3) Closed head injury with contusion and/or intracerebral haemorrhage (see p. 201).
(4) Encephalitis.

The picture of neurological disability in all the above will depend upon the site of maximal cortical involvement. In addition, the primary cerebral damage will give rise to secondary vasomotor paralysis with congestion and oedema of the brain. This will produce a downward displacement of the cerebral hemispheres leading to diencephalic and brainstem compression, which we describe in Part B below.

Part B: Involvement of diencephalic and brainstem-activating centres

The diencephalon and brainstem may be affected:

(1) as a result of brainstem compression:

   (i)   from above,
   (ii) from the side (uncal herniation),
   (iii) from below; or

Table 6 Localisation of brainstem involvement (see text for full explanation)

	Diencephalic		Uncal	Midbrain and upper pons	Lower pons and upper medulla	Lower medulla
	Upper	Lower				
Response to pain	Appropriately directed	Abnormal flexor	Appropriately directed	Abnormal extensor	Nil	Nil
Pupils	Small with intact light reflex	Small with intact light reflex	Unilateral and then bilateral dilatation	3–5 mm irregular	3–5 mm and unresponsive	Dilated and unresponsive
Eye movements	Full (rolling)	Full	Third nerve palsy	Hard to elicit internuclear ophthalmoplegia	Absent	Absent
Respirations	Eupnoeic Cheyne–Stokes	Eupnoeic	Eupnoeic	Tachypnoeic	Shallow 20–40/min	Slow and irregular
Other	Grasp reflexes	—	Development of ipsilateral hemiplegia	Diabetes insipidus	—	Falling arterial pressure
Ocular vestibular (ice-water calorics)	Deviation of both eyes to side of lesion			Adducting eye fails to move across the midline	Absent	Absent
Oculocervical (doll's head manoeuvre)	Normal (see text)			Adducting eye fails to move across the midline	Absent	Absent

(2) as a result of direct injury.

Brainstem compression

The initial symptoms are often focal and relate to the specific site of the supratentorial lesion. So there may be evidence of headache, focal neurological signs or symptoms, or a strikingly asymmetrical neurological examination. The evolution over time to unconsciousness will depend on the rate of brain expansion, and may vary from hours to weeks. The expanding brain will progressively compress the neuraxis, the hallmark of such compression being evidence of a progressive involvement of lower brainstem centres—termed rostrocaudal deterioration.

As indicated, the expanding cortex may impinge upon the brainstem either from directly above or from the side.

(1) From above, pressing the brainstem directly downwards. The early stages are marked by predominant involvement of the diencephalon, as outlined below and also in Table 6.

    (i)   Eupnoeic respirations which may be interrupted by sighs or yawns or by Cheyne–Stokes breathing.

    (ii) Appropriately directed response to pain, for example supraorbital pressure.

    (iii) The grasp reflex, elicited by firm palmar pressure, emerges.

    (iv) Relative lack of brainstem involvement.

        (a) Eye movements are intact, seen spontaneously as rolling eye movements or in response to doll's head manoeuvre or ice-water calorics (see below).

The doll's head manoeuvre is carried out by observing the effect on eye movements of briskly and fully rotating the head on the neck and trunk (if necessary, whilst the patient is temporarily disconnected from the ventilator). In normal people the eyes will stay looking forward whilst the head is moved, whereas in abnormals, the eyes will move in the same axis as the head.

Ice-water calorics are carried out as follows. First, inspect the external auditory canal to ensure the tympanic membrane is intact and, if necessary, remove wax. Lift the head if possible to 30° to the horizontal. Using a thin catheter inserted into the external auditory canal, slowly instil up to 50 ml of ice-cold water whilst observing the eye movements. In a conscious patient this is extremely uncomfortable, for it induces severe vertigo, nausea and vomiting, together with nystagmus of which the fast component is away from the irrigated ear. In the unconscious patient with an intact brainstem, the response obtained is of tonic conjugate deviation of the eyes towards the irrigated ear. Having tested one side, 5 min should elapse before testing the other in order to allow the currents induced in the semicircular canals to subside.

(b) The pupils are usually small, but careful examination with a bright light (and if necessary hand lens or ophthalmoscope) discloses an intact light reflex.

(v) With further diencephalic compression, the directed response to pain is replaced by abnormal flexor posturing of the arms with extension of the legs—so-called decorticate rigidity.

The importance of recognising this stage of diencephalic compression is that if the cause of the compression can be treated effectively (as, for example, oedema may) full recovery is likely. Further caudal involvement usually involves infarction, implying increasing morbidity and mortality (see Table 6).

Later stages, due to continuing compression, and leading to involvement of the midbrain and upper pons are indicated when the following events occur.

(i) Cheyne–Stokes respirations are replaced by tachypnoea

(ii) Abnormal extensor postures of the arms with pronation of the forearms are evoked by pain—'decerebrate' rigidity.

(iii) The pupils dilate moderately to 3–5 mm and are frequently irregular.

(iv) Eye movements in response to doll's head manoeuvre and ice-water calorics become harder to elicit. The adducting eye may fail to move past the mid position (internuclear ophthalmoplegia).

The lower pons—upper medulla stage—is reached when the following occur.

(i) The respirations become shallow at 20–40 per min.

(ii)   The pupils stay at mid position (3–5 mm) but do not respond to light.

(iii) Eye movements in response to the doll's head manouevre and ice-water calorics become unobtainable.

(iv)   There is no response to pain arising from the trigeminal area.

Terminally, with medullary involvements:

(i)   the respiration slows and becomes irregular;

(ii)   the arterial pressure falls with a variably slow or fast heart rate.

(2) Pressure on the brainstem from the side—uncal herniation. This is usually caused by expanding masses in the middle fossa (including the temporal lobe) which compress the brainstem laterally. The diencephalon may be little involved initially; the third nerve almost invariably is. Thus, a unilaterally dilating pupil is accompanied by a level of consciousness which may vary from alertness to coma.

Once the pupil dilates fully, oculomotor involvement follows and ice water calorics reveal full third nerve impairment (failure of the eye to move from full abduction and downward deviation). All eye movement becomes lost as ichaemia spreads to the midbrain. Frequently the opposite cerebral peduncle becomes compressed against the tentorial edge, and a hemiplegia ipsilateral to the original lesion becomes added to the contralateral hemiplegia which frequently preceded it. Posturing in response to pain may be flexor but is usually extensor in the arm.

With involvement of the midbrain and upper pons, the opposite pupil may become fixed in mid position, and may also dilate widely. As with downward central compression, respiration becomes hyperpnoeic, extraocular movements become increasingly difficult to elicit, and bilateral extensor posturing emerges.

(3) Finally, brainstem compression from below may arise from expanding subtentorial masses. These may either be intrinsic to the brainstem, destroying the reticular activating system, or extrinsic, compressing it. Extrinsic lesions, in addition, may cause the cerebellum to herniate upwards through the tentorial notch, compressing the upper brainstem and diencephalon, and/or downwards through the foramen magnum, compressing the medulla.

The hallmark of this category of patients therefore is evidence of pontine or midbrain damage at the onset of coma. Further clues for a subtentorial lesion include a history of occipital headaches, vertigo diplopia and/or vomiting at the onset of coma.

Initially, therefore, before frank upward herniation, if there is compression of the middle third of the pons, the patient is usually drowsy rather than comatose, with constricted (1–2 mm) but reactive pupils and lateral rather than vertical ophthalmoplegia. Nystagmus if present, is gaze paretic; respirations are initially unaffected but may later become ataxic and then slow; corticospinal tract signs and mild limb ataxia usually emerge.

As upward cerebellar herniation proceeds, signs of midbrain compression evolve (see Table 6) with extensor posturing, unequal mid position fixed pupils with either failure of upward elevation of the eyes or frank downward conjugate deviation.

Downward herniation of the cerebellar tonsils may be suspected by resistance to neck flexion or spontaneous opisthotonic posturing but if sufficiently advanced is obviously a terminal event, with respiratory and circulatory collapse ensuing shortly thereafter.

Direct injury to the brainstem

Direct injury to the brainstem gives rise to focal neurological signs which depend on the actual site of the lesion, and which can be inferred from Table 6. Typically, the signs may be fairly restricted and frequently asymmetrical, thus providing accurate localisation

(1) Midbrain lesions, if centrally placed, interrupt both the light reflex pathways and frequently oculomotor interconnections Thus, pupils are mid position and fixed with either nuclear or internuclear (see above) ophthalmoplegia, and bilateral frequently asymmetrical corticospinal tract signs.

(2) Upper and midpontine involvement is marked by small reactive pupils, a gaze palsy to the side of the lesion and sometimes evidence of fifth (absent corneal) or seventh (lower motor neuron facial asymmetry) nerve involvement.

(3) Lower pons lesions similarly have small reactive pupils with lateral eye movements absent, but vertical eye movements spared (vertical doll's head manoeuvre). There may be flaccid quadriplegia, or alternatively abnormal extensor posturing The respiratory rhythm is frequently interrupted with cluster apneustic or ataxic patterns.

If cerebellar and brainstem signs are elicited, the possibility cerebellar haemorrhage (p. 194) must not be forgotten. Cerebellar infarcts accompanied by developing oedema may also behave like an expanding mass lesion and are similarly susceptible to potentially life-saving neurosurgical decompression.

Part C: Metabolic encephalopathy

There are a number of features which distinguish metabolic encephalopathy from the previously discussed structural causes of coma.

(1) Coma is nearly always preceded by an interval of decreased awareness, impaired cognitive function and personality disturbance.

(2) Even when other brainstem functions are lost with depression of consciousness, absent ice-water caloric reflexes and abnormal extensor posturing, the pupillary light reflex is usually preserved. This simultaneous involvement of many levels of the neuraxis with relative sparing of some functions at the same level is typical of metabolic encephalopathy. Progressive rostrocaudal deterioration (see above) does not occur.

(3) Abnormal movements typical of metabolic encephalopathy include a fine tremor at 8–10 Hz, bilateral asterixis (frequently found in, but not confined to, hepatic encephalopathy), and multifocal myoclonic jerks.

Sustained focal neurological deficits are usually absent. However, there are two exceptions to this rule which can be a trap.

(i) Hypoglycaemic hemiplegias which may completely resolve with prompt and adequate treatment (p. 172). Similar findings have been reported in hepatic coma, uraemia and hypernatraemia.

(ii) Although lateral conjugate deviation of the eyes strongly suggests a structural lesion, downward conjugate deviation may be caused by metabolic disturbance— particularly certain drug overdoses.

(4) Your examination will include smelling the breath (diabetic ketoacidosis, uraemic fetor, fetor hepaticus and alcohol) and testing for neck stiffness (meningitis, subarachnoid haemorrhage and tonsilar herniation).

Part D: Psychogenic unresponsiveness

There are several features of this state which resolve diagnostic confusion.

(1) The eyelids are usually held firmly shut, resist opening and, when released, snap shut. The slow passive closure of the lids of the comatose patient is rarely successfully reproduced.

(2) The corneal reflex evoked by blowing or by a wisp of cotton-wool is rarely successfully suppressed. Similarly, tickling the eyelashes usually evokes eyelid twitching.

(3) Roving or disconjugate eye movements exclude this diagnosis.

(4) Ice-water calorics evoke nystagmus, the normal response, rather than tonic deviation. This physical sign is unequivocal and diagnostic.

MANAGEMENT OF THE UNCONSCIOUS PATIENT

Evaluation of the evolution and patterns of neurological deficit should have enabled you to make a sophisticated guess at the site and nature of the lesion. However, common to all the categories are a number of basic considerations which, in rough order of priority, are as follows.

(1) Assure oxygenation. This is quantified by measuring arterial gases or minute volume (more than 4 l/min usually indicates adequate ventilation). Clear blood and vomit from the pharynx by suction. If ventilation still seems inadequate, intubate and ventilate, otherwise turn your patient into the semirecumbent coma position. If there is a history of neck pain or trauma, do not extend the neck to intubate. Obtain a lateral neck x-ray without moving the patient. Rarely, an emergency tracheostomy may be necessary. Cardiac arrhythmias, provoked by intubation, may be prevented by atropine 0.6 mg i.v. beforehand. Remember that inhalation of gastric contents is a frequent problem in patients who have lost their protective reflexes (see p. 96).

(2) Maintain circulation. If there is a vasomotor paresis from brain stem involvement or inadequate intake from prior illness, the effective circulating volume may be low. Infuse fluid in the usual way with CVP control (see p. 343). If the circulating volume is adequate, as judged by the CVP response, it may be necessary to infuse dopamine (see p. 300).

(3) Hypoglycaemia should be checked using BM stix, sup

plemented if you obtain a low reading by a formal blood glucose. This should be done while (1) and (2) are going on.

(4) Fits. Other than brief minor motor episodes, these should be controlled (see p. 210).

(5) If there is evidence of mass lesion (focal neurological signs and/or signs of raised intracranial pressure), start treatment for raised intracranial pressure with a bolus of mannitol and controlled hyperventilation (see p. 205). Obtain a CT scan; do **not** do a lumbar puncture.

(6) If there is evidence of metabolic disorder, send blood for: electrolytes and urea; osmolality; blood gases; calcium; and glucose. Save blood for toxic screen, liver function tests, coagulation studies, thyroid and adrenal function, blood culture and initial viral titre. If examining a traveller recently arrived from the tropics, consider cerebral malaria, yellow fever, typhoid and typhus. Obtain a CT scan and, in the absence of focal swelling, do a lumbar puncture.

(7) Check the rectal temperature. Extremes of temperature should be corrected (see pp. 265 and 271).

(8) If there is a history of alcoholism, or if there is ophthalmoplegia, or if i.v. dextrose is to be infused, give thiamine 100 mg i.v. beforehand to prevent or treat Wernicke's encephalopathy.

(9) If you suspect a narcotic overdose, give naloxone 0.4 mg every 5 min until the patient arouses (see p. 72). If there is evidence of narcotic addiction (look for needle marks), dilute 0.4 mg in 10 ml of diluent and inject slowly to avoid precipitating an acute withdrawal crisis.

(10) If coma is interrupted by agitation, small (5 mg), preferably i.v., doses of diazepam should suffice.

(11) General care of the unconscious patient includes the following.

   (i)   Attention to pressure points (a pillow between the arms, 2-hourly turning, perhaps a ripple mattress). Obviously, bed linen must be frequently changed if it becomes soaked with urine or stained with faeces.

   (ii)   In the absence of spontaneous blinking, avoid exposure keratitis by methylcellulose eyedrops, and, if necessary, securing the eyelids with adhesive tape.

   (iii) Urinary incontinence can frequently be managed satisfactorily with a sheath urinal for a man, but for women an indwelling silastic catheter, inserted with strict attention to asepsis, is the most satisfactory solution.

Part E: Flow diagram of coma management

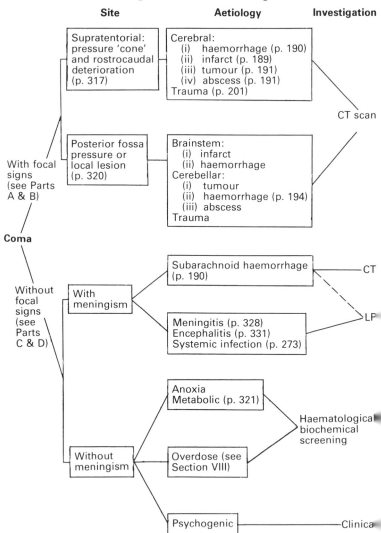

REFERENCES

1   Bates D. (1985). Predicting recovery from medical coma. *Br. J. Hosp. Med.*; **May:** 276.
2   Bates D. (1985). Management of the comatose patient. *Hosp. Update*; **June:** 425.
3   Cartlidge N. E. F. (1979). Clinical aspects of coma—the assessment of acute brain failure. *Trends in Neurosci.*; **2:** 126.
4   Leader (1981). Outcome of non-traumatic coma. *Br. Med. J.*; **283:** 3.
5   Plum F., Posner J. B. (1982). *The Diagnosis of Stupor and Coma.* Philadelphia: F. A. Davis.

Severe chest pain[1]

DIAGNOSIS

Consider the following sites.

- *The heart*
  Angina.
  Myocardial infarction (see p. 10).
  Cardiac arrhythmias (see p. 23).
  Pericarditis—the pain is often affected by posture, and is usually worse lying down. It is also promptly relieved by indomethacin.
- *The lungs*
  Pneumonia (see p. 99) and other causes of pleurisy.
  Pulmonary embolus (see p. 47).
  Pneumothorax (see p. 80).
  Carcinoma of the lung.
- *The oesophagus*
  Oesophagitis, with or without hiatus hernia.
  Oesophageal achalasia.
  Ruptured oesophagus—this gives rise to mediastinal emphysema thus you may feel crepitus at the root of the neck.
  Oesophageal carcinoma.
- *The aorta*
  Dissecting aneurysm (see p. 58).
- *The mediastinum*
  Mediastinitis.
  Mediastinal pneumothorax.
- *The nerves*
  Cervical spondylitis or other causes of root compression.
  Herpes zoster—you will be vindicated should a characteristic rash appear.
- *The abdomen*
  Acute cholecystitis.
  Acute exacerbation or perforation of a peptic ulcer.
  Pancreatitis (see p. 116).
- *Thoracic wall*
  An almost endless list of conditions involving muscles, bone nerves, etc., of which perhaps the commonest is an unexplained sharp pain over the precordium, lasting a few moments, called 'precordial catch'.

MANAGEMENT

The possibilities can usually be reduced to two or three by a careful history and examination.

However, it is wise always to ask for:

(1) an ECG,
(2) a chest x-ray,

and if in doubt, observe the patient in hospital, bearing in mind that a normal ECG does not exclude a myocardial infarction.

REFERENCE

1   Lichstein E. *et al*. (1973). Evaluation of acute chest pain. *Med. Clin. N. Am.*; **57**: 1481.

Severe headaches

The commonest cause of severe headache is migraine. Usually there is a preceding history of episodic throbbing headaches, associated with nausea and photophobia. Classically, visual symptoms such as teichopsia may precede or accompany the headache. Neck stiffness from concomitant muscle spasms, photophobia, and transient focal signs (see p. 192) may mimic meningitis which must, in cases of doubt, be excluded by examination of the CSF.

Other, more serious causes of headache which constitute emergencies are as follows.

(1) Meningitis.[2,8] This has four cardinal signs: headache, stiff neck, photophobia and fever. However, they may all be absent. A lumbar puncture is indicated if two of the four are present. It may also present as drowsiness, confusion, convulsions, focal neurological signs or coma. In the immunologically uncompromised host, three organisms account for most cases of bacterial meningitis: *Neisseria meningitidis* (a gram-negative coccus causing meningococcal meningitis, usually affecting young adults and invariably sensitive to penicillin) *Haemophilus influenzae* (a gram-negative rod usually found in the under fives, and usually sensitive to chloramphenicol), and *Streptococcus pneumoniae* (a gram-positive coccus causing pneumoccal meningitis, the prominent organism in the elderly and, except in rare, geographically discrete instances, sensitive to penicillin).

The organism may be identified by direct staining of CSF. However, where no organisms can be seen, for example in partially treated meningitis, distinguishing antigens may rapidly be identified after counterimmune electrophoresis.[6]

Until positive identification is secure, give drugs as indicated below.

(i) To children above 8 years and to adults: benzylpenicilli 1.2–2.4 g i.v. in divided doses at 4-hourly intervals, on th presumption that they will be harbouring the meningo coccus or pneumococcus.

(ii) To children below 8 years: penicillin G 250 000 U/kg pe day in divided doses 4-hourly i.v., plus chloramphenico

100 mg/kg per day i.v. in divided doses at 6-hourly intervals.

(iii) In cases of penicillin allergy or anxiety about the use of chloramphenicol: cefuroxime 3 g 8-hourly (children 60–75 mg/kg 8-hourly) can be used. As this antibiotic has a satisfactory action against all three above organisms, some authorities recommend it as first-line therapy.

When the organism is identified, proceed as follows.

(i) Meningococcal meningitis: benzylpenicillin is the drug of choice, given as above. If i.v. therapy becomes technically difficult and the organism is sensitive to sulphonamides, these may be given orally instead. Prophylaxis, either as rifampicin 10 mg/kg every 12 h for four doses, or, if the organism in sulphonamide-sensitive, sulphadimidine 500 mg 6-hourly for eight doses, should be offered to intimate contacts of your patient.[5]

(ii) Pneumococcal meningitis: again, give benzylpenicillin as above.

(iii) *Haemophilus influenzae*: chloramphenicol is now the drug of choice. Previously, ampicillin 300 mg/kg per day i.v. in divided doses given 6-hourly was advocated. This has now been precluded by the rapid rise in incidence of ampicillin resistance. Cefuroxime is an effective alternative to chloramphenicol. Rifampicin 20 mg/kg per day for 4 days should be given to any contacts under the age of 4 years.[5]

Triple therapy with penicillin, sulphonamide, and chloramphenicol, intrathecal antibiotics, and steroids are unnecessary in treating meningitis caused by these organisms.

Differentiation from other causes of meningitis rests on examination and culture of the CSF.

(i) Tuberculous meningitis.[4] This may present with a few weeks history of increasing headaches, malaise and drowsiness, or have a more acute course of seizures, focal signs and progressive obtundation. Evidence of tuberculous infection elsewhere may be lacking, but the tuberculin skin test is usually positive. All cases of suspected meningitis should have CSF examined and cultured for TB organisms since, although the CSF cell response is typically lymphocytic, occasionally polymorphs may predominate. Recommended therapy is isoniazid 10–15 mg/kg per day (plus pyridoxine 50 mg/day) with rifampicin 600 mg/day and either ethambutol 25 mg/kg per day or pyrazinamide (0.5 g t.i.d.).

(ii) Cryptococcal meningitis. This is not uncommon in America and is not confined to the diabetic or otherwise immunologically compromised. History is similar to that for tuberculous meningitis and likewise may be acute or more insidious. Diagnosis is made by India-ink microscopy of the CSF and examination for cryptococcal antigens. Recommended therapy is a combination of amphotericin and flucytosine, in the same dosage as for candidal septicaemia (see p. 311).

(iii) Amoebic meningitis. This is usually identified only when apparently pyogenic meningitis fails to respond to conventional therapy since the amoeba in CSF resembles white cells. Recommended therapy is amphotericin B 20 mg/day or, if the organism is a *Hartmanella* species, sulphadiazine 100 mg/kg per day given as 6-hourly doses i.v.

Unusual organisms may cause meningitis in immunologically compromised people, and in neonates. Discussion of treatment in these cases is beyond the scope of this book.

(2) Subarachnoid haemorrhage (see p. 190).

(3) Giant cell arteritis.[1] This condition commonly causes headache by involvement of the medium-sized arteries of the scalp or dura, and is virtually unheard of below the age of 55 years. In about half the cases, involvement of the central retinal artery causes blindness which usually occurs between 1 and 3 months after the onset of the headaches. However, transient or permanent amblyopia may be the presenting symptom. In the typical case, the superficial arteries are tender, swollen and often pulseless. The ESR is usually above 60 mm/h.

Occasionally, superficial arteries are not clinically involved and the ESR is normal. Where the history is suggestive, a length of temporal artery when examined serially may show the characteristic histology. High doses of steroids, e.g. 60 mg of prednisone per day, should be given immediately the diagnosis is suspected.

(4) Hypertensive encephalopathy (see p. 44).

(5) Herpes simplex encephalitis.[3] Here the headache is accompanied by 3–4 days of increasing irritability, confusion, neck stiffness and, in the later stages, occasional seizures followed by progressive stupor. Percussion of the skull may demonstrate lateralised tenderness. The CSF shows lymphocytosis, raised protein count and characteristically increased red cells. Typically, temporal lobe involvement may be demonstrated by focal signs and symptoms and EEG abnormalities, radionuclide scan and CT scan changes. However, herpes encephalitis may be more generalised or focal elsewhere.

Herpes simplex vesicles are rarely found on lips, skin or genitalia, but where present virions may be identified by electron microscopy of vesicle fluid. Failing this positive diagnosis, treatment as outlined below should be given to any patient with encephalitis and focal clinical features, on the presumption that they have herpes simplex encephalitis. The diagnosis may be confirmed retrospectively by a rising antibody titre to the herpes virus. Treatment, with i.v. acyclovir 10 mg/kg 8-hourly for 10 days, has reduced the mortality to 19% at 6 months.

(6) Subdural haematoma (see p. 191).

(7) Pituitary apoplexy (see p. 167).[7]

REFERENCES

1   Cullen J. F. (1976). Ophthalmic complications of giant cell arteritis. *Surv. Ophthalmol.*; **20**: 247.

2   Lambert H. P. (1983). The treatment of bacterial meningitis. *Br. Med. J.*; **286**: 741.

3   Leader (1986). Herpes simplex encephalitis. *Lancet*; **i**: 535.

4   Lehrich J. R. (1982). Tuberculous meningitis. *N. Engl. J. Med.*; **306**: 91.

5   Nelson J. D. (1982). How preventable is bacterial meningitis? *N. Engl. J. Med.*; **307**: 1265.

6   Peltola H. O. (1982). C-reactive proteins for the rapid monitoring of infections of the central nervous system. *Lancet*; **i**: 980.

7   Riskind P. N. (1986). A case of pituitary apoplexy. *N. Engl. J. Med.*; **314**: 229.

8   Schwartz M. N. (1984). Bacterial meningitis: more involved than just the meninges. *N. Engl. J. Med.*; **311**: 912.

The acutely painful joint

DIAGNOSIS

Your main objective in dealing with an acutely painful joint is to exclude infection, as the consequences of delayed treatment of an infective arthropathy are disastrous.

(1) A septic arthritis gives rise to an acutely tender, swollen, reddened, hot, immobile joint (all the classical features of inflammation—calor, dolor, rubor and laesio functio—are present). There is usually only a single joint involved, although a preceding flitting arthropathy is common in gonococcal arthritis. Here skin lesions, usually small papules on the trunk or limbs, and tenosynovitis are also common; 80% have positive genitourinary cultures, and this gram-negative coccus is the commonest infecting organism in the 16–40 age group. The frequency of other organisms in non-gonococcal infective arthritis is presented in Table 7.

(2) Joint infection usually occurs via haematogenous spread: 50% of patients have an obvious source for their infection, pneumonia, skin sepsis and gonorrhoea being the most common; 80% are pyrexial, although rigors are uncommon.

Chronic joint disease, prosthetic joints, intra-articular injections, contiguous osteomyelitis or a deep wound all predispose toward joint infection.

(3) Other possible causes of an acutely inflamed joint or conditions that may cause confusion are as follows.

    (i) Crystal arthropathy, either gout or pseudogout. The crystals can be found in the joint fluid.

Table 7 Organisms in non-gonococcal infective arthritis

Organism	Frequency (%)	Gram staining characteristics
Staphylococcus aureus	68	Gram-positive coccus
Streptococcus	20	Gram-positive coccus
Haemophilus influenzae	1	Gram-negative bacillus
Gram-negative bacilli (various)	10	

(ii) An inflammatory monoarthritis, usually a seronegative arthropathy in association with Reiter's disease, inflammatory bowel disease, psoriasis and occasionally with rheumatoid, SLE or rheumatic fever. Evidence for the associated disease will usually be present.

(iii) Osteomyelitis. Here the pain is over the bone, rather than the joint.

(iv) Superficial cellulitis. The features of inflammation will be present, but joint movement will be relatively preserved, and the area of skin redness not necessarily locally confined to the joint.

(v) Haemorrhagic arthritis. Although pain and loss of function are prominent, other features of inflammation are not, and a history of trauma or bleeding disorders is usual.

(vi) An acute episode supervening on chronic joint disease, usually rheumatoid arthritis. However, here, if only one joint is involved, infection must be excluded as the cause (see above).

The above considerations should help with the diagnosis.

(4) The key investigation is joint aspiration and analysis of the synovial fluid (Table 8). Aspiration should be considered in any swollen joint where there is the faintest possibility of infection.

Table 8   Analysis of synovial fluid

	Bacterial infection	Non-bacterial inflammation
Total leucocyte count	50 000–200 000 cells/mm³	>20 000 cells/mm³
	>90% polymorphs	<50% polymorphs
Sugar	Low in 50% of cases	Usually normal—occasionally low in rheumatoid
Gram stain	positive in 70%	negative
Culture of joint fluid	positive in the majority	negative
Crystal	negative	positive in gout (uric acid) and pseudogout (calcium pyrophosphate)
Blood	negative	positive in haemorrhagic effusions

Fifty per cent of patients have a total peripheral blood white cell count above 10 000/ml and 50% have positive blood cultures, both of which tests should therefore be undertaken.

(5) X-rays. These usually show non-specific soft tissue swelling, and are not immediately helpful.

MANAGEMENT

(1) Drainage. Repeated large-bore needle aspiration, draining the joint completely, should be performed, twice daily if necessary.

(2) Antibiotics. There is no need for intra-articular antibiotics. Intravenous antibiotics should be used. If the gram stain is positive, be guided by this. If negative, give i.v. penicillin 2 mega units 6-hourly to the sexually active 16–40 year old and a combination of gentamicin (see p. 310) and penicillin to other patients.

(3) Joint rest. In the acute phase the joint should be immobilised in an optimal functional position with a splint. Passive movement should be started as soon as pain allows.

(4) If the joint is inaccessible (as the hip), you should consult with your orthopaedic surgical colleagues, as operative aspiration and drainage will probably be required.

FURTHER READING

Goldenberg D. L., Reed J. I. (1985). Bacterial arthritis. *N. Engl. J. Med.*; **312:** 764.

The acutely breathless patient

Consider the following causes.

(1) Left ventricular failure (see p. 39).
(2) Pulmonary embolus (see p. 47).
(3) Mitral stenosis (see p. 41).
(4) Cardiac tamponade (see p. 60).
(5) Asthma (see p. 75).
(6) Acute respiratory tract infections (see p. 99).
(7) Pneumothorax (see p. 80).
(8) Large pleural effusion (see p. 89).
(9) Acute upper airways obstruction (see p. 86).
(10) Massive pulmonary collapse (see p. 84).
(11) Myasthenia (see p. 218).
(12) Acute infective polyneuritis (see p. 215).
(13) Overdose of salicylates, dinitrophenol or sulphanilamide (see p. 242).
(14) Overbreathing ostensibly due to anxiety (often called 'hysterical' overventilation).

OVERBREATHING DUE TO ANXIETY

Diagnosis

(1) This usually occurs in young women. The overbreathing may be far from obvious to the casual observer.
(2) The history is nearly always classical: first they felt breathless; then they had tingling, first around the mouth, then in the arms and legs; then they had cramps of the hands which took up the main d'accoucheur position. If sufficiently prolonged, the patient may lose consciousness.
(3) You must aim to establish the sequence of events. In this condition, anxiety precedes breathlessness, whereas in the other causes of breathlessness, the converse is usually the case.

Management

1) Emergency treatment is to persuade the patient to breathe in

335

and out of a paper bag. This allows them to rebreathe their CO_2, lowers the pH, reverses the alkalosis and relieves the tetany. This relieves most of the tension and is accompanied by massive verbal reassurance and, if necessary, sedation with 50 mg of chlorpromazine or 10 mg of diazepam.

(2) Do not leave it at that—try to establish the precipitating cause. Their anxiety may be due to a somatic or psychiatric condition for which they may need help.

(3) Do not forget that anxious overbreathing young women may also have taken an overdose of salicylates. Always test the urine.

In other states such as diabetic ketosis, the uraemic syndrome, and encephalitis, the patient is obviously breathing abnormally deeply but this is rarely attended by the distress which accompanies the above condition.

Social problems

Some people who arrive at casualty departments, including those listed below, turn out to be unable to provide for themselves and are often referred to the medical team.

(1) The frail elderly patient who does not require admission on strictly medical grounds.
(2) The patient who comes to casualty with a trivial illness, but is of no fixed abode.
(3) The mother who, as a result of contracting a minor illness, is unable to cope at home because of poor circumstances and innumerable children.
(4) The psychiatric patient who needs in-patient treatment, but will not come in.

The basic requirements enabling an individual to fend for himself are:

(i)   food,
(ii) money,
(iii) shelter and clothes,
(iv) companionship—in its widest sense,
(v)   mental stability (to the extent that they will harm neither themselves nor other people) and the ability to manage (i) to (iv).

Help to provide for these requirements may be forthcoming from the following sources.

(1) Your hospital social worker, who should always be contacted first if possible.
(2) If you do not have one, or the problem arises at night and the social worker is unavailable, your local authority Social Services Department should provide a 24 h social work service. Ring their duty officer for advice on the problems which may need dealing with.

(i)   Psychiatric problems. It is clearly wise to avail yourself of any local psychiatric help first, either within your hospital or from the area mental hospital, but this may not always be forthcoming. In any case you may need a social worker

to help you to commit to hospital a patient against his wil
under the appropriate section of the Mental Health Act.

(ii) Problems with children. Your hospital may provide
facilities for admitting young children with their mother
If not, it may be necessary that they be taken into care via
the Social Services Department.

(iii) The elderly. If the advice of a geriatrician is not easily
available, social work advice re domiciliary service
and/or residential accommodation is essential.

(3) Many areas have hostels run by the Department of Health and
Social Security (DHSS), social services, or voluntary organisations, e.g. the Salvation Army, for people of no fixed abode
Your casualty department has the telephone number of these
hostels, which, however, are under no obligation to tak
people. The DHSS should provide for each area an emergenc
office which is open in the evenings for emergency payments c
provision of hostel vouchers.

(4) The patient's general practitioner (if he has one) will be able t
provide valuable background information and should be con
tacted, if available.

(5) There are various voluntary organisations, e.g. the Samaritan
who provide a 24 h supportive service for those in acute distre
(for example potential suicides) or other similar organ
isations—Alcoholics Anonymous, Depressives Anonymou
Gingerbread (mainly daytime).

(6) The police carry 'place of safety warrants' (for children and th
mentally ill) and are a source of information re local hostels.

If these organisations cannot immediately help, the person shou
be admitted to hospital pro tem.

Central venous pressure and pulmonary artery occlusion catheter (Swan–Ganz)

Central venous pressure [1,4,5,9]

Central venous pressure measurements play an important role in many medical emergencies and now comprise a standard technique in which careful attention to detail is necessary for reliable results to be obtained.

TECHNIQUE [1]

(1) Your objective is to introduce an i.v. catheter into the superior vena cava. So introduce an i.v. catheter into a vein which will give you ready access to the superior vena cava. This is preferably done percutaneously or, if necessary, by cutting down on the vein and introducing the catheter under direct vision. The vein most often used is the median cubital or basilic vein, though any vein which has ready access to the superior vena cava may be used, for example the external or internal jugular or subclavian.

Difficulty may be experienced negotiating the section of the basilic vein where it passes under the clavipectoral fascia. This may be overcome by twisting the catheter so that its natural lie is in the line of the vein, by abducting the arm to a right-angle and externally rotating it, or by passing the catheter onwards while at the same time infusing fluid through it, thus displacing the walls of the vein. The position of the catheter **must** be checked after insertion by x-ray. If it is in the superior vena cava, the level should rise and fall a few millimetres with expiration and inspiration. If it does not:

    (i)   it is not in a vein;
    (ii)   you are not far enough up the vein;
    (iii) the tip is angled against the vein wall—withdraw slightly;
    (iv) the catheter is partially blocked—flush out with 5 ml of sodium citrate;
    (v)   the catheter tip is in the right ventricle—the level is suspiciously high and pulsatile.

(2) The catheter is connected by a three-way stopcock to a water manometer. The scale should be zeroed against a fixed refer-

ence point on the patient who should, therefore, always be in the same position when the measurements are taken. The following values all apply to the horizontal patient lying supine.

Reference point	*Normal values*
5 cm dorsal from angle of Louis	1 to 8 cm
The angle of Louis	-4 to $+3$ cm

The reference point of 10 cm above the surface on which the patient is lying is not acceptable.

INTERPRETATION

(1) The measurement obtained reflects at least four variables:

    (i)   intrathoracic pressure;
    (ii)   efficiency of the right heart;
    (iii) venous tone; and
    (iv) volume of venous blood.

It may appear surprising, therefore, that useful results can be obtained at all. These variables are examined in more detail below.

- The gentle oscillation associated with respiration which was noted above, reflects change in the intrathoracic pressure.
- The efficiency of the right heart should not be compromised unless the circulation is being overloaded or there is myocardial disease. However, it is vital to remember that the CVP measures right atrial pressure and often fails to reflect left atrial pressure, particularly in the presence of myocardial disease. In these circumstances a patient may develop severe left ventricular failure without altering the CVP, so a pulmonary artery pressure line (with facilities for measuring pulmonary wedge pressure) should be set up wherever this is available (see p. 346).
- The fact that venous tone cannot be measured in the clinical situation neither refutes its existence nor diminishes its importance. The capitance of the circulation is controlled by venous tone, which is therefore a primary influence upon CVP as a measure of the volume of venous blood. Venous tone is increased, for instance, by both catecholamine infusion and haemorrhagic shock. In these clinical circumstances, a relatively high CVP may be more a reflection of raised venous tone than of adequate blood volume.
- In normal circumstances, the venous system is readily distensible; venous tone may relax to the extent that a substantial increase of blood volume may produce no change in CVP. For these reasons a

single recording of CVP is unlikely to be helpful in assessing and monitoring the replacement of blood volume. A series of readings is more likely to be informative, particularly if they are taken in response to rapid but small increments in blood volume. Specifically, if 200 ml of fluid is infused over 2 min, we recognise three patterns of response (Fig. 24).

(i) A persistent rise of more than 3 cmH$_2$O can be taken to exclude hypovolaemia and probably implies hypervolaemia (pattern a).

(ii) A rise of 2–3 cmH$_2$O during the infusion with return to the baseline at 15–20 min is characteristic of normovolaemia (pattern b).

(iii) A rise of 2–3 cmH$_2$O during the infusion with return to the baseline within 5 min is highly suggestive of hypovolaemia (pattern c).

(2) An initial reading of the CVP which is well within the normal range should not put you off performing this diagnostic/therapeutic test because, as mentioned above, a high venous tone may raise the CVP and mask hypovolaemia.

(3) If hypovolaemia is suspected on clinical grounds, careful expansion of the circulating volume with the CVP maintained a few centimetres above normal (but less than 10 cm above the angle of Louis, otherwise pulmonary oedema may be precipitated) should be tried. For details of which fluids to infuse, see p. 299. This may actually cause a slow fall of CVP by inducing relaxation of the veins, and allow infusion of more fluid. This

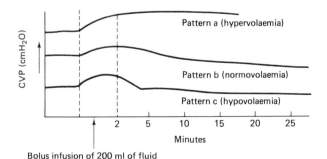

Fig. 24 Central venous pressure patterns of response to 200 ml of fluid infused over 2 min.

gradual fall in CVP may also be observed in response to both vasodilators and steroids, or if an infusion of pressor amines is stopped.

(4) Where hypovolaemia has been confirmed, infuse fluid rapidly until the CVP rises into the upper half of the normal range. If this level is maintained for several hours, the patient will become warmer and pinker, and will start to look better. A satisfactory urine output may also be restored (but be on your guard for acute renal failure, see p. 142). It is now reasonable to run the infusion at a slower rate and allow the CVP to fall. Should the CVP drop below normal, full fluid repletion has not taken place and an infusion rate sufficient to keep the CVP in the midnormal range is required. The deleterious effects of hypovolaemia are due to poor tissue perfusion. Although a low cardiac output is usually the primary cause of poor perfusion, the subsequent hypoxia produces locally and centrally mediated responses in the peripheral vasculature which aggravate the situation (see p. 296). Typically, there is: (a) arteriolar constriction producing a further reduction in tissue flow; and (b) venular dilatation which pools blood in the periphery reducing venous return and therefore cardiac output. Clearly the longer a patient remains hypovolaemic, the more firmly this vicious circle becomes established. For this reason the consequences of prolonged hypovolaemia can only be reversed by maintaining the CVP within or above the upper range of normal for several hours. Large volumes of up to 15–20 litres may be required and can only be given safely with a reliable CVP line. Any excess of water and electrolytes may be excreted after normal homeostasis has been restored without harmful effects.

OTHER USES

(1) In conditions where the problem concerns myocardial efficiency rather than hypovolaemia (e.g. myocardial infarction), a rise in CVP may give warning of impending heart failure. Remember that in these circumstances the CVP may not reflect left ventricular function, and that in any case a CVP line is no more than a jugular venous pulse with a college education.

(2) A sudden fall in the CVP in a patient with suspected gastrointestinal bleeding may herald further blood loss before this becomes clinically apparent (see p. 107).

(3) Prolonged i.v. feeding is only possible through a CVP line.
(4) Blood samples may be withdrawn through a CVP line providing 20 ml is withdrawn first (and of course rejected) to clear the dead space.

COMPLICATIONS [2]

Although CVP measurements are of enormous help in situations of hypovolaemia, and to a lesser extent myocardial infarction, venous catheters may be associated with complications and they should not therefore be used unless a definite therapeutic advantage is expected. The following complications have all been recorded.

(1) Thrombophlebitis. This is almost inevitable if the catheter is left in for more than 10 days and is probably due to mechanical irritation. The inflammation is rapidly settled by short-wave therapy but a blocked vein is inevitable and occasionally oedema of the upper arm results.
(2) Infection of the cut-down site.[8] This is minimised by scrupulous aseptic technique and Polybactrin spray. It is also a good idea to separate the sites of entry of the catheter through the skin and into the vein as far as possible.
(3) Infection of the catheter tip is less easily avoided and may give rise to septicaemia. At any rate, it is a wise precaution to culture the catheter tip after it has been removed.
(4) Erosion of the vein. If this is not recognised early, it may cause widespread infusion of fluid into subcutaneous tissues, which is painful for the patient and may be dangerous if secondary infection occurs. If suspected, the catheter should be withdrawn.
(5) Arterial bleeding sufficient to cause tracheal obstruction is a potential complication of all jugular and subclavian puncture techniques.
(6) Pneumothorax is a specific complication of subclavian vein puncture.
(7) Catheter embolus into the right heart is known to occur if the catheter is inadvertently broken at the site of entry to the skin. Surgical advice should be sought.

REFERENCES

(see p. 351).

The pulmonary artery occlusion (Swan–Ganz) catheter[1,3,6,9]

PULMONARY WEDGE PRESSURE

(1) Knowledge of the left and right atrial pressures is essential:

    (i)   for the informed management of complicated acute right or left heart failure;

    (ii)   to help the assessment of hypovolaemia, and thence the amount of fluid replacement required, in any critically ill patient; this is particularly useful if there is heart disease, when the usual relationship between the right and left atrial pressure may not obtain (see p. 14);

    (iii) to distinguish between non-cardiac and cardiac pulmonary oedema (see p. 40).

(2) It is also wise to have an arterial cannula for continuous monitoring of pressure and for blood gas analysis. Finally, cardiac output measurement, available if you use a catheter with a thermodilution facility, provides all the information necessary to manage the most complex haemodynamic problems.

THE SWAN–GANZ CATHETER

Right atrial pressure is measured with a CVP line (see p. 341), whilst left atrial pressure is most conveniently measured using a flow-directed pulmonary artery catheter (Swan–Ganz catheter). This can be put in at the bedside without x-ray control. The left atrial pressure at which pulmonary oedema will appear is dependent on the serum albumin as an approximate index of the COP (see p. 298). A simple formula expresses the interrelationship of serum albumin and the development of pulmonary oedema (see p. 39).

The catheter

This has two lumens, one of which controls a balloon immediately behind the catheter tip, while the other opens a single end-hole. The balloon has a dual function: during insertion it is blown up (with air or CO_2—make sure you know the correct amount) as soon as the catheter tip is in the right atrium. (The junction of the superior vena cava and the right atrium is at 15–20 cm from the usual insertion point—the internal jugular vein.) Thereafter the balloon acts as a sail, directing the catheter tip in the direction of maximal flow, i.e. through the tricuspid and pulmonary valves. Once the tip is in a small pulmonary artery, inflation of the balloon will occlude the artery proximally, leaving the end-hole exposed to the pulmonary capillary pressure (pulmonary wedge pressure), which is assumed to be identical with left atrial pressure.

Swan–Ganz catheters are usually available in two sizes:

7F with a 1.5 cm³ balloon
5F with a 0.8 cm³ balloon

We have found the larger size easier to manipulate and less likely to clot.

For cardiac output measurement, using the thermodilution technique, catheters are available with an additional injection lumen in the right atrium and two thermistors beyond, so you can also use most catheters to measure CVP.

Catheter insertion

This is best done by an antecubital cut down on the basilic vein—a technique free of serious complications. Alternatively, the catheter can be put into a large central vessel, usually the internal jugular, percutaneously. 7F catheters require a guide-wire technique; we use Desselet insertion sheaths. Remember to use a sheath one size larger than the catheter to allow for the deflated balloon. 5F catheters can be passed through large cannulae, e.g. a 12G medicut, but a guide-wire technique is probably safer.

(1) Advance the catheter into the vein—say 10 cm—and connect to the transducer (see Measurement below).
(2) Blow up the balloon when the tip is in a central vein, preferably just at the junction of the vein and right atrium.
(3) Advance slowly, allowing the catheter tip to be guided by flow. Except in conditions of very low flow, it is usually easy to cross the valves. If there is trouble crossing the pulmonary valve, it is worth trying the balloon both deflated and inflated to get across. Sometimes loops form in the right atrium which makes

manipulation difficult. Withdraw the catheter with the balloon blown up in order to straighten it out.

(4) Try to find a position which gives a good pulmonary artery tracing with the balloon deflated (Fig. 25b) and a good wedge pressure with it inflated (Fig. 25c). The right ventricular pressure tracing (Fig. 25a) is shown for comparison.

(5) X-ray the chest.

Measurement

The exact set-up will vary with the equipment available. Most equipment designed for continuous monitoring is precalibrated such that a given pressure change produces a set deflection on the scale. It therefore only remains to zero the transducer to atmospheric pressure. Some equipment may require both zero and calibration adjustments, in which case it is necessary to adjust the calibration using a mercury column.

(1) The catheter is connected via a manometer line, a three-way tap and an Intraflo continuous flushing device to the transducer. The Intraflo is also connected to a pressure bag containing N saline and 500 units heparin.

(2) As the transducer is set up, exclude all air bubbles from the system.

(3) To zero the transducer, follow the steps below.

    (i)   Close the tap between catheter and transducer (if this is not done, blood will flow back up the catheter into the transducer dome).

    (ii) Open the tap on the side arm of the transducer to air.

    (iii) Adjust the tracing on the monitor to zero.

    (iv) Close the transducer side arm and open the transducer to the catheter. Zero the transducer after it has warmed up—this will take about 30 min. Remember that the wave form used for catheter positioning does not have to be quantitatively accurate; we ordinarily put the catheter in first and then zero (and calibrate if necessary) afterwards.

    (v) You should, of course, take expert advice if you are not familiar with these practicalities.

(4) Recordings are made:

    (i)   with the patient flat;

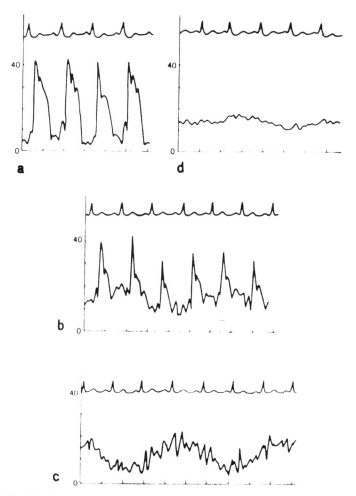

Fig. 25   Pressure tracings from the right heart. **(a)** Right ventricle. **(b)** Pulmonary artery. **(c)** Pulmonary artery wedge pressure. **(d)** Damped wedge pressure tracing. The pressure scale is in mmHg. The paper speed is 25 mm/s with 10 mm spaces shown. The baseline variation in the tracings is due to the effect of respiration. An ECG recording is also displayed.

(ii)   with the transducer at the level of the angle of Louis or midchest (see CVP, p. 342)—this is most important;

(iii)   of phasic and then mean pulmonary wedge pressure. The phasic nature of the recording is due to the pressure swings related to respiration, and it is the mean pulmonary wedge pressure which you should act on. (Many monitors produce a digital display of systolic, diastolic and mean pressures.)

(5) Before acting on a single or serial recording, it is essential to check their validity, by checking the following.

(i)   Mechanical factors, such as the level of the transducer and the zero level.

(ii)   That there is a recognisable wave form (see p. 349).

(iii) That there is respiratory variation of the wave form.

(iv)   That the pulmonary artery trace returns on deflation of the balloon.

(v)   The pulmonary capillary wedge pressure should be less than the pulmonary artery pressure (see below).

If you have any reason to disbelieve the calibration of a preset machine, it is easy to attach a manometer line to the transducer side arm and produce a vertical column of water (13.5 cmH$_2$O = 10 mmHg). Important decisions may be made on the basis of differences of less than 4 mmHg in the wedge pressure, that is 20% of the upper limit of normal. It is easy to make errors of this order in recording.

Problems

(1) 'Overwedging'. Sometimes the catheter tip is lodged in a small pulmonary artery whose diameter is less than that of the balloon. As the balloon is blown up, a wedge tracing appears and starts climbing continuously. If this happens, deflate the balloon, pull it back and then fill it slowly again, stopping as soon as the wedge appears. Make sure the trace rises and falls with respiration.

(2) Failure to wedge. Try repositioning the catheter. Alternatively, pulmonary artery diastolic pressure usually approximates to wedge pressure.

(3) Damped trace (see Fig. 25d) and blocked catheters. This is the major problem with continuous monitoring.

(i)   Check that there is no air in the system and that the transducer is not open both to air and to the patient.
(ii) Try flushing the catheter using the fast flush mechanism on the Intraflo.
(iii) Try a hand flush. Use a 1 ml syringe—being of narrow bore, this generates the highest pressures. Make sure you flush only the catheter and not the transducer. Be careful not to introduce any air.

The catheter is more likely to block while the balloon is inflated. For this reason, flush the catheter after each reading. If the trace does become damped, it is important to try to clear it as soon as possible otherwise the catheter will become blocked.

(4) Positive end expiratory pressure (PEEP). Remember PEEP will add to the intrathoracic pressure and that PA and wedge recordings will be accordingly higher.

Complications

These are infrequent.[7]

(1) As in the insertion of any central line, damage to the lung or large arteries may occur. It is wise to do a chest x-ray after inserting the catheter.
(2) Arrhythmias related to the passage of the catheter may occur, and will require a standard therapeutic approach (see p. 23).
(3) The line may be a source of infection. It should be inserted with scrupulous aseptic technique, and removed as soon as possible.[8]
(4) Pulmonary infarction is a hazard, particularly if there is persistent wedging of the catheter.
(5) Air embolism is said to be a hazard, which can be overcome by filling the balloon with CO_2.

REFERENCES

1 Davies J. M. (1982). Cardiovascular problems. *Hosp. Update*; **Nov.:** 1359.
2 Dunbar R. D. *et al*. (1981). Aberrant location of central venous catheters. *Lancet*; **i:** 711.
3 George R. J. D., Banks R. A. (1983). Bedside measurement of capillary wedge pressure. *Br. J. Hosp. Med*.; **March:** 286.

4   Latimer R. D. (1971). Central venous catheterisation. *Br. J. Hosp. Med.*; **5:** 309.
5   Leader (1974). Jugular venous pressure. *Br. Med. J.*; **4:** 367.
6   Leader (1978). Swan–Ganz catheter. *Lancet*; **ii:** 357.
7   Leader (1983). Complications of pulmonary artery balloon flotation catheters. *Lancet*; **i:** 37.
8   Maki D. G., Goldman D. A., Thame F. S. (1973). Infection control in intravenous therapy. *Ann. Intern. Med.*; **79:** 867.
9   Shaver J. A. (1983). Hemodynamic monitoring in the critically ill. *N. Engl. J. Med.*; **308:** 277.

Index

Note: numbers in bold type indicate main page reference

The publishers and authors want to ensure that *Medical Emergencies* continues to be an invaluable aid for the house physician. If you have any comments or suggestions for incorporation in the next edition, please write to:

Heinemann Medical Books, Halley Court, Jordan Hill, Oxford OX2 8EJ

Turn the page for news of other titles in the series